# The Unlikely Marathoner

*How to conquer your big goals and run with it!*

Donna Campisi

First published by Busybird Publishing 2017
Copyright © 2017 Donna Campisi

ISBN
Print: 978-1-925585-66-7
Ebook: 978-1-925585-67-4

Donna Campisi has asserted her right under the Copyright, Designs and Patents Act 1988 to be identified as the author of this work. The information in this book is based on the author's experiences and opinions. The publisher specifically disclaims responsibility for any adverse consequences, which may result from use of the information contained herein. Permission to use information has been sought by the author. Any breaches will be rectified in further editions of the book.

All rights reserved. No part of this publication may be reproduced, stored in or introduced into a retrieval system, or transmitted in any form, or by any means (electronic, mechanical, photocopying, recording or otherwise) without the prior written permission of the author. Any person who does any unauthorised act in relation to this publication may be liable to criminal prosecution and civil claims for damages. Enquiries should be made through the publisher.

**Cover image**: Kev Howlett and Scott McNaughton
**Cover design:** Busybird Publishing
**Layout and typesetting**: Busybird Publishing
**Editor**: Beau Hillier

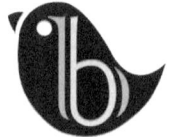

Busybird Publishing
2/118 Para Road
Montmorency, Victoria
Australia 3094
www.busybird.com.au

"What can I say? Donna is a true inspiration and ray of sunshine. The ability to overcome such adversities with a permanent smile is truly mind blowing. Donna is a huge role model for all youngsters, and if only more people were like her our world would be a much better place."

> Sam Maguire
> *Sam's Run for Cancer.*

"When I am speaking publicly I always say to take two words out of your vocabulary: 'can't and never'. Reading Donna's book, you really do learn that there is no such word as 'can't'! This book will help you learn that anything really is possible and Donna's story is proof of that. I believe that after reading Donna's book you will be ready to really reach within yourself to work out what your own dream goal is and have the commitment to achieve it."

> Carol Cooke AM
> *Athlete, Author and Speaker*

"When I interviewed Donna for *Runner's World* a few years ago, I knew as soon as she opened her mouth that she was a force to be reckoned with. She's equipped with an iron will and a fierce determination to push past any obstacle that's thrown at her. If you want to reach a goal, any goal, Donna will help you get there."

> Sabrina Rogers-Anderson
> *Writer and Author*

"Donna is an absolute inspiration – she has put together her insights and method of how she does what she does in this book. It's simple and easy when you know how to achieve any goal that you set. Absorb this information but more importantly take massive action. Donna truly holds the key to success and your dreams coming to reality."

> Natasa Denman
> *Ultimate 48 Hour Author*

# Dedication

To my parents, Nata and Vince, who are both amazing people. Their love, strength, courage, compassion, encouragement, prayers, patience and resilience have been an amazing gift, I feel truly blessed. Thank you, thank you!

It's difficult to put into words the true gratitude I have for the support, love, patience, empathy, strength and motivation that I received from my 'fellow soldier' during the tough battles we faced and endured together. The times of uncertainty in RCH and the treatment and rehabilitation afterward were the most difficult challenges I've had to endure. A *big* thank you to my mum. You inspire me every day and were my reason to never give up through the tough battles!

# Contents

| | |
|---|---|
| Foreword by Pat Farmer | i |
| Introduction – Ready! Set! Go! | iii |
| Chapter 1 – Conquering 'I Can't' | 1 |
| Chapter 2 – Choosing Your Distance | 19 |
| Chapter 3 – Finding Your Core | 29 |
| Chapter 4 – Commitment Gives Power | 37 |
| Chapter 5 – Jump Right Out | 43 |
| Chapter 6 – Training Buddies | 55 |
| Chapter 7 – Mental Roadblocks | 63 |
| Chapter 8 – Celebrating the Journey | 77 |
| Chapter 9 – Obstacle Challenge | 83 |
| Chapter 10 – Winning Language | 101 |
| Chapter 11 – Your Roadmap to the Finish Line | 115 |
| Chapter 12 – The Baby Step Method | 135 |
| Afterword | 141 |
| Acknowledgements | 151 |
| About the Author | 155 |
| Turn Dreams into Reality | 159 |
| Donna as a Speaker | 161 |
| Adventure Beyond Limits | 165 |

# Foreword

# by Pat Farmer

At the tender age of seven, Donna's life was thrown into chaos. Like a country unwillingly drawn into war and the night eclipsing the day, a veil of confusion and uncertainty cloaked her and those she loved.

The war that her body waged against her seemed so unfair for someone so young, yet even in this most fragile state, she showed the courage of a veteran soldier – a trait that would inspire all those who know her and read her story.

Donna has fought for every breath and every step. She reminds us of the steel locked within us all and encourages us to find our way through the obstacle course of life and to achieve our dream.

The marathon is a wonderful analogy for life. You start starry-eyed with dreams of grand success but shortly into the journey, you are hit with a curve ball, something that throws you off course from completely out of left field. You need to decide if the goal is worth the pain. Somehow, you draw strength from past experience and push through. As a taunt or a reward, life grants you a second wind.

Things are good again but nothing worthwhile is ever easy – and so a little further on down the track, usually around the 30 km mark, you hit a wall. Just like a crash test dummy, you're thrown around and pulled inside out.

If your purpose and motive is great enough then you will soon realise that in this life, even the tough times don't last forever. So you hang in there and just over 42 km after you set off, you cross the finish line. You discover that with hard work and a will of iron, with the right people as support, nothing is impossible.

Donna uses the struggle of completing her own marathon to show all of us that life and living life is the Holy Grail. If Donna can endure all that she has and make life a success, then what are we all waiting for? Get out there and live!

> Hon Pat Farmer AM
> – Ultra-athlete, author of *Pole to Pole*, and friend
> 1 February 2017

# Introduction

# Ready! Set! Go!

*The Unlikely Marathoner* is for those who want to achieve their *big* hairy scary goals that seem more like a dream than an actual reality. You *can*!

This book will guide you to reach your goals in work and play, in business and in your personal life. I will lead you through these chapters and help you plan a Baby Step Method that works, so you can conquer your big goal and run with it.

We all have big dreams, but only a small percentage of people go through the full journey to achieve their dreams. Why? Because it seems too scary, crazy and difficult to most people!

I will share my insights, frustrations, experiences, excitement, lessons and my Baby Step Method in this book for you to use, so you can gain knowledge of how to conquer your big scary goals and run with it!

'You should write a book, Donna!' I've heard this many times. Whenever I've mentioned my story to people, or after a speaking event, they are always surprised and amazed when they hear of my past and the goals I've achieved.

Others who've known me for some time now, or even all my life, have been amazed at the outcome of my journey, and I am truly grateful for their love and support.

So here it is at last: *The Unlikely Marathoner*. I initially started writing this book as an autobiography, but then realised that I've always wanted to use my story to inspire and encourage others to help reach their goals – so I changed my direction a little.

I still share moments of my life, such as my experience of surviving a stroke when I was only seven years old. I like to call them training sessions in life, which include my more recent challenge of learning to run again.

But please note, this is not aimed solely at people with running goals; this book is for any *big* goal that you want to achieve.

Enjoy!

## Background

To begin this journey with you, I need to share with you a background of my story so you can understand the experiences I have had – and the insights, trainings and lessons I will share throughout this book.

### #training #lesson
### November 1978 – My life-changing moment

My story begins as an ill seven year old child, not far off turning eight. First I developed severe diarrhoea, which resolved, but then one week later I had a dry cough, fever, headache, abdominal pain, vomiting and what looked like a purple rash on the bottom of my right foot (at the time we didn't know this was from a burst vein). I had been treated with antibiotics, as I wasn't resting well and my temperature was high. After a few visits to the doctor and a diagnosis of tonsillitis, I still wasn't improving. I had these symptoms for a week.

Then it happened!

Like a frightening alarm, my parents woke up in the early hours of the morning to see my small thin body convulsing. This had never happened before. I had wet the bed, my whole body was shaking and my eyes were going in every direction. My parents were in shock at what they were witnessing! I was unable to respond to their reactions or control what was happening to my body.

I was rushed to my local hospital; after doing a number of tests, the medics admitted they'd never seen this before and didn't know what was wrong. They flew my mum and me to the Royal Children's Hospital in Melbourne; as an emergency patient, there was no time to waste. My father and brother drove over 500 km from Mildura to Melbourne with no idea of what they'd find at the end of their lengthy trip.

We arrived at the Royal Children's Hospital with a whole team attending to me. They did test after test, but they seemed bewildered – they called me 'The Mystery Girl'.

Eventually there was a diagnosis: right hemiparesis. The right side of my body was immobile from a haemorrhage in the left side of my brain. The haemorrhage and the purpuric lesions on the right foot were thought to be secondary to a mycotic embolus (infected aneurysm). Other findings included meningitis, staphylococcal septicaemia, splenomegaly and endocarditis, which indicated a prolapsing mitral valve – including a hole in my heart and a heart murmur. I had anaemia (iron deficiency), osteomyelitis of my right ankle bones and aphasia (loss of speech). Doctors predicted I'd never walk or talk again, and announced to my parents that I was lucky to be alive.

With constant rehabilitation, determination, strength and support from family and medical professionals – and maybe even my own stubbornness at times – I then became known as 'The Miracle Girl' with the team at RCH.

I left the hospital eventually; although still needing a wheelchair most times, I could walk with support and callipers on – but still slow and unsteady, needing the aid of a quad cane. My right hand and arm were still a problem and I needed more therapy, as I was only able to perform simple tasks with special aids when I left the RCH.

I now walk confidently with a leg brace that helps me with my foot drop, and changed from being right handed to left handed. I can live a life independently doing most things.

Later, at fourteen years of age, I made another visit to the RCH in a critical condition. I was diagnosed with type 1 diabetes, and I now need to inject insulin every day. But I'm alive and here to tell my story.

As my mother always said to me when I was eight, 'Donna, there's always someone worse off than you.' Not really wanting to think that, as I really didn't want to think there was *anyone* going through a more difficult time, I knew what she meant and felt grateful for surviving the stroke. I felt safe with the strength of my mum beside me every day ... even if there were tough times ahead.

I have never seen my mother give into hopelessness. This I truly admire her for. The strength that she even shows to this day never differs from all those years ago.

My strength today is an adaptation that not only comes from my own life experiences, especially through this chapter of my life. But also comes from my mother who showed me strength each day. I'm forever grateful for that.

These I consider my early days of training for my journey ahead in life.

*'Life's challenges are not supposed to paralyse you; they're supposed to help you discover who you are.'*
 – Bernice Johnson Reagon

## #training #lesson
## October 2012 – Planting the seed

In supporting my friend Eleni, I attended her time management workshop in 2012. During the workshop, Eleni asked the group, 'What would you do if you had more time in your day?' Her eyes glanced around the room and stopped at me – I was up first.

I had just been for a walk that weekend, for the first time in too long! I lived across the road from a beautiful beach and had parks nearby with walking tracks. I thought to myself, *I should do this more often*. I did once upon a time, and I even drove to the beach for a scenic walk back then – and now I had it right outside my doorstep!

My response to Eleni: 'I would take more time to exercise, like I used to.' There, I said it out aloud!

What was stopping me? Nothing! All I had to do was prioritise, rearrange my time, get out there and enjoy the environment around me. I did this sporadically, not really setting a routine.

My life was at a stage where I really needed to set a routine for my manic misplaced lifestyle, full of goals but not getting anywhere. Was it that I had too many goals and doing too many things at once, never really moving forward? I felt like I was on a treadmill going through all the motions but getting nowhere in particular! Maybe this was because they weren't really my true heartfelt goals? Perhaps I wasn't focused on what I really wanted.

Looking back at that time, I seemed to be

following suggestions, ideas, and goals of what others thought I should do, and I felt that I could 'make it work'. I was working so hard, achieving the small steps along the way, but nothing lined up with what I was truly about. It was exhausting!

I've always been a passionate person and found that when I follow my passions and what I truly believe in, this is where I succeed the most. This was the time for me to reflect and work out where I needed to spend my time more, and where I could spend less time doing things that needed less or no attention.

*'If you want to make good use of your time, you've got to know what's most important and then give it all you've got.'*
   – Lee Iacocca

### #training #lesson
### November 2012 – The first step

Although I was enthusiastic about most people in my life at the time, this was a wakeup call for me spending time on *me*.

I needed to move for a moment away from my desk and take time out to enjoy walking the path. To see the trees, the green grass, the blue sky and fluffy white clouds; to feel the sun on my skin; to experience the energy of the people relishing the spring weather … this was the time-out I needed to realise there was more to life than working for and servicing someone else's motivation, rather than my own.

It officially started on 16 November 2012. I stepped off the treadmill of 'going through the daily motions' and went out for a walk on a real path, making some 'me time'. On this day, I chose to re-prioritise my steps and my actions, by taking on board my new time management plan. But little did I know where this 'me time' would take me.

It was only a few years before that someone asked me, 'What can't you do since having a stroke, Donna?' I needed time to think, as I'd never been asked this question and always liked to try to focus on what I *can* do, rather than what I *can't*.

My response: 'I haven't had the confidence to run since the stroke. In fact, the last time I remember running was when I was seven!' At that moment, without me even realising, a seed was planted.

So, on this particular sunset evening, walking along the beach, I noticed the super-fit bodies that swooped past me in their smooth running motion, and some not-so-smooth bodies that looked worn out. I wondered silently, *Why don't I give this running thing a go?*

So there I was, walking on a concrete path with nobody to catch me. *What if I fall?* I thought. *Well, you've done that plenty of times, when walking! So what?*

Agreeing with the second voice in my head, I held my breath like I were about to jump into the sea, as if somehow that would help me in my revived attempt at running. I made the leap and went for it. This was something I hadn't done on my own in thirty-four years.

I counted my hobbling steps as I moved hesitantly forward: one, two, three ... making it to twenty steps, I felt the need to stop and breathe. Pleased with myself for surviving the twenty steps without kissing the concrete, I was excited for my second attempt, wanting to improve on that number.

Twenty-four was my next successful attempt; this time I remembered to breathe on step fifteen. *Woo hoo, an improvement!*

Next was twenty-five reasonable steps. I was safe! I just needed to practise and I knew I would improve every day!

The last attempt for the evening was a triumphant thirty puffed-out steps! Although this may sound lame to the average person, I accepted long ago that I'm not the average person.

That evening in my adventurous forty-five minute walk, all sorts of ideas came to my overly enthusiastic mind. I thought perhaps I could organise a fundraiser fun run, while wondering if I could learn to run again. Could I possibly get some help and run 4 km – is that too big of a goal for me? Hey, I was gradually improving from twenty steps to thirty! Surely I could push myself to reach 4 km. *Hmmm, I wonder ...*

To cut a long story short, 4 km turned into 42.2 km. Yes, you read it right. My goal to learn to run again looked like this: someone who hadn't ran for thirty-four years due to a stroke, and only able to run thirty tentative steps, made a goal to run in the Melbourne Marathon in eleven months' time! This was huge for me, a *big* scary goal that seemed unachievable. This was where Run Donna Run began, as a personal challenge for me, raising funds for the RCH and encouraging others that *there's no such thing as can't*.

But this book is not just about me and my crazy 'stroke to marathon' story. I'll be sharing my stories and lessons learned along the way, but this is about how you can achieve your big goal too – and I'm not just talking about running.

Let's do it. Ready! Set! Go!

# Chapter 1

# Conquering 'I Can't'

All too often the words 'I can't' can easily fall out of our mouths. If said too often, it can become an embedded belief that will never get you to that big goal you dream about.

When you take this belief out of your mind, then you gain confidence and the courage to achieve.

If we keep saying, 'I can't', we actually tend to believe it after a while and the people around us do too; they're not going to expect big things out of you, and neither are you!

Instead, we can create a habit to ask ourselves, 'How can I?'

Have you ever noticed when someone asks you, 'Can you do this?' You're either going to say yes or no. It's just a one-word answer, isn't it?

What if someone asked, 'How can you?' These words are great! It's an interesting question to ask, because it actually makes you think instead of just saying yes or no. It's easy to say no and it's easy to make excuses – but, 'How can I? How can I do this? How can I do that? How can I achieve my big scary goal?' This is what it's all about.

If there's a big goal that you've been dreaming about and you've been either too scared or allowed someone to put it in your mind that it's crazy, I understand. I've been there.

Through my experiences and what I have achieved, I'll share my insights, not just from what I've achieved, but also from the struggles and tough times that I've had as well. It hasn't all been sunshine and lollipops, as they say.

Here, we're going to learn new things about ourselves. When asking yourself, 'Can I? Is it possible?' a lot of people make excuses. Often it's either time or money stopping people achieving their big goals.

Sound familiar? I've had those reasons too, believe me. But then I stopped to think, 'Okay, surely I can find another way. How can I possibly afford to do this? How can I find the time to do this?'

Two great questions. To find a solution, you need to think outside the box.

The thing is, if you ask yourself 'can I' instead of 'how can I', you're always going to dream; you'll never achieve that big goal and live with regret until the day you die.

We don't want this to happen. This is why you're reading this book right now. I really want to help you by sharing my experiences, insights and steps for you to achieve your big, scary goal.

Moving past the 'I can't,' is an important mind shift to achieving your goal. Believing you can is the first step when beginning the Baby Step Method to achieve your goals.

This was evident with my marathon challenge – which seemed like a crazy idea at first, but I had to put it in my mind that nothing could stop me from doing it. Even though I could easily come up with so many excuses, I wasn't going to be that person.

*'Whether you think you can, or you think you can't, you're right.'*
   – Henry Ford

### #training #lesson
### November 2012 – The first meeting

Returning home from my adventurous walk, with my attempt at running thirty steps, I remembered meeting a guy at a business seminar I'd attended, only a month before.

I attended a seminar and sat down in the front row with a friend and another man beside me whom I didn't know. During the presentation, we were asked by the speaker to participate in a five minute exercise by turning to someone we hadn't met, introducing ourselves and telling each other what we did as a profession.

We all stood up and I turned to the man beside me, a thin tall stranger with a huge smile. We exchanged our introductions, and then he told me about the running business he owned with a business partner, where they coached people on how to run properly and avoid injury as well as giving them the right nutrition advice.

I was enthralled and quickly shared my story – from my stroke to where I was at that moment, and how I had found running a challenge since I was seven. Our five minutes went fast, so I asked for his card to look them up, which he didn't have, so he wrote his website on one of my notepads. That was the last time we spoke, as we had a break and I didn't see him after that.

So that night a month after the seminar, I raced straight to my pile of notes, trying to find which notepad he scribbled his website on.

I panicked at the thought that I may have misplaced that particular piece of paper; I couldn't even remember the name of the guy who wrote his details for me, let alone his business name. But then I finally found it – phew!

I liked what I read on their website; I thought these guys sounded like they had the experience and knowledge to help me, even though this body of mine is not your usual body to work with. I liked the sound of this coaching team.

Shaun was a sports musculoskeletal therapist; I didn't know fully what that meant, but it sounded impressive and it also stated he was an exercise physiologist.

Chris, I noticed by the photo, was the guy I'd met. His bio described him has having a keen interest in nutrition and other performance enhancements – this sounded interesting. They had both completed marathons and crazy ultra-marathons and raised funds for charity while doing so. I liked these guys already!

My next step involved an attempt to write a very impressive email to get these guys on my side – to coach me to run. With their help I could do a fun run – maybe a 4 km fun run, that would be awesome! I thought this while questioning myself if it was even doable.

After carefully writing the hopeful email (then editing and re-editing and reading it another ten times), I confidently clicked the send button at 10.06 pm, happy with what I proposed and hoping for a positive response.

Exactly twenty-eight minutes after I clicked the send button, I received a reply email from Shaun.

> 16/11/2012, at 10.34 PM
>
> *Hi Donna,*
>
> *Let's do it!*
>
> *I'll call you tomorrow to discuss it further.*
>
> *It would be our pleasure to help you and the thousands of people that you will help.*
>
> *Looking forward to working with you.*
>
> *Shaun*

I loved this dude's enthusiasm, but I wondered at the same time if he should be discussing this with his business partner first. I hadn't even met this Shaun guy yet!

The next day I received an email from Chris, sounding keen too. Excellent!

*17/11/2012, at 12.40 PM*

*Hi Donna,*

*I actually remember you telling me about your stroke and thought you had such a positive outlook on things.*

*I was hoping you would look us up, and I agree, this would definitely be a win-win situation for all of us on so many levels.*

*Look forward to catching up soon.*

*Chris*

Soon my phone rang as well. 'Hello?'

'Hi Donna, this is Shaun.' This calm, deep, professional sounding voice was the sports musculoskeletal therapist, exercise physiologist and running coach, calling me just as he said he would the previous evening.

'Oh, thanks for calling,' I replied, trying not to sound too surprised. This guy was actually enthusiastic and managed to respond like he said – and on a weekend!

We chatted for a while. I was uncertain where I was going to take this, although I knew I wanted to raise funds for the Royal Children's Hospital and encourage others at the same time.

'Thanks for agreeing to coach me to run again! I really appreciate your help. I was thinking I could do a fundraiser with my new goal of running, maybe a 4 km run. Do you think you could help me run that distance? Do you think that's possible?'

I enquired. I felt enthusiastic but also silently hesitant, trying to think what that distance would be like on foot … running. It's just a number, but I remember being able to do a 4 km walk-a-thon many years ago for a fundraiser, very determined as a child in my new calliper.

'Yes, you could do that distance!' he claimed confidently. This guy hadn't even seen me walk yet, let alone my attempt at running thirty tentative steps. He sounded too confident to me. 'Donna, you need to do something big though. If you want to raise funds and create an impact, and encourage and inspire others, you need to run more than 4 km. Anyone can do that. You should run a marathon, Donna!'

What? Was this guy crazy?

'How about the Melbourne Marathon in October?'

'A marathon? You haven't even seen me walk, let alone run! A marathon is huge!' Was this Shaun guy crazy? What was he thinking? *Who does he think I am, some superhero? Maybe he is, but I'm only just starting to run! A marathon?*

'Donna, anyone can run a marathon, it's all to do with your mindset.'

I paused and I wondered if he could hear my mind ticking. I had heard this before; I knew what he was talking about. I'd heard similar words used in the past when it came to goal-setting, but this was different, this was massive … this was a freakin' marathon!

'Let's catch up and meet in person and we can talk further about it. You don't have to decide anything yet.' This guy was serious – it wasn't a passing idea that just fell out of his mouth.

'Okay, that sounds great! Will this include Chris too? I would like to catch up with both of you,' I said in a fake pleasant voice, hoping that Chris would slap him around and help him see 'the light'.

In the meantime, from 17 to 26 November 2012, I kept practising my own style of running, after the evening of my first scary thirty step attempt. I went out for a half hour each evening: walking, running a few steps, walking, then running a few steps more, repeating this process until I felt I could go no more.

It was hard, but I stayed out for the half hour as my walking took me places with no issues, except for the usual limp that has been with me for the past thirty-four years. The limp has improved to a point that I have become used to it, without feeling uncomfortable when people are obvious with their stare. I now walk with a confident limp, smiling as I write this, not allowing other people's reactions to bother me anymore.

*'If you walk confidently in the direction of your dreams and dare to live the life which you have imagined, you will meet with a success.'*
   – Henry David Thoreau

Focusing on your goal and not allowing other things to get in your way is a major path to success. But things in life will get in your way – that's just life. Further on in this book I'll talk about how you can get past that, and move past those reasons for stopping your big goal. We can come up with plenty of reasons to say, 'This is all too hard, I can't do this.'

But you're reading this because you don't want to be that person. You could ask, 'What if I fall, what if I trip up?' That's part of the journey. It's okay to stumble. Just get back up again. I've stumbled plenty of times, literally and mentally, but it's okay.

People stumble and then say, 'It's too hard,' and don't bother picking themselves up again. That's where I find there's a real loss of potential – a loss of achieving something that could have been huge, something great that would have made that person into who they want to be, instead of holding this great dream in their mind that they don't think they could ever achieve.

It's also very common for people to question themselves with, 'What will other people say? What if they laugh or doubt my decision?' I could tell you a number of stories of people laughing, calling me crazy, doubting me; some people who were really close to my heart were doing this, even if just out of concern. There were also other people laughing and thinking I was crazy for having a goal to run again. They just didn't see my marathon challenge as a possibility. We've got to try to ignore those people around us.

Sometimes it's people around us who you feel you can't ignore. But I'll talk in an upcoming chapter about how to keep focused and about the importance of the people you surround yourself with. This is very important when reaching big goals, so stick with me and stay on track.

Believing you can is the first important step. This was an important lesson I learned when going through rehabilitation after surviving my stroke.

### #training #lesson
### 1979 – Julie's mantra

'Donna, there's no such thing as can't!' Julie announced confidently with a stern voice as my hands and knees stayed glued to the gym mat.

Julie had never spoken like this before, in such a stern voice!

I loved Julie, my physiotherapist; she was a fun bubbly woman who supported me through my rehab. I thought Julie was awesome! I loved going to the physio department every day because I would see Julie and her smile. I had been seeing Julie every day since I was able to get out of bed and into a wheelchair.

But this was a day when I really did not like Julie!

In my physio session on this particular morning, Julie asked me to do a new 'trick' that I was too scared to do.

Julie carried me out of my wheelchair and onto the grey gym mat, placing me on my hands and knees. This was a task for both of us to get right, peeling my fingers out to support my right hand and stiff curled wrist. My right fingers always wanted to curl under, especially when we tried to straighten my wrist. I managed to place my hand in a proper position to support my arm and help me balance. Julie supported me by kneeling beside me.

*Chapter 1 – Conquering 'I Can't'*

There I was, on my hands and knees in a crawling position; at this point I'd been unable to crawl or walk since I had been at RCH. I had never been asked to try this new challenge, until now.

'Donna, today I want you to try to crawl. What you need to do is move one hand forward and the opposite knee forward at the same time. I'll be here to support you. Are you ready?'

'I can't!' I pleaded with Julie, thinking this was the most difficult and ridiculous thing she had asked me to do so far.

'If you don't try, you won't know,' Julie responded. 'I will be here to support you.'

'But I can't!' I hoped that she would help me get back into my own special wheelchair so I could race as fast as I could out of the PT department, never to be put onto the gym mat in a position of vulnerability again. 'I can't!'

'Donna, I'm right beside you. You are safe. Just give this a go,' continued Julie.

'I can't! I can't!' I pleaded with tears rolling down my cheeks.

Julie was normally the fun lady with a smiley badge and big blue eyes that were so vibrant, I sometimes found myself staring with amazement and awe. Today she wasn't the fun, jolly lady whose cheerful laugh I always looked forward to hearing. How could this be?

She was as stubborn as me!

Finally Julie said to me, after many attempts to encourage me to move, 'Donna, there's no such thing as can't!' I looked at her strangely as she said it again. 'There's no such thing as can't!'

Stopping my sobs, feeling puzzled, I thought: *Yes, there is! I've heard this word before, I'm sure it's a word in the dictionary! What is she saying?* Back to my sobbing, I looked up to Julie, pleading with desperation. 'I can't!'

Still not wanting to help me back into my safe wheelchair, Julie walked to the door, stating again, 'Donna, there's no such thing as can't,' and walked out of the room, leaving me on my hands and knees on the gym mat – all by myself.

The room was closing in on me. I felt a rush of emotions fill my entire body: fear, anxiety, helplessness, and vulnerability. I stayed on my hands and knees, too afraid to move a scrawny limb, with tears flowing down my cheeks and hitting the grey gym mat. Julie was no longer beside me to support my body if I fell. But I could no longer keep still, shaking with my deep gasps between uncontrollable sobs, trying so hard to hold back my blubbing, knowing that Julie was watching me through the little window on the door. I tried so hard to keep my balance and calm down to catch my breath.

I had difficulty spreading my fingers out on the mat, while holding my wrist firm to keep me up and steady; my fingers wanted to curl into a claw.

Finally I calmed down, stopping my sobs and taking deep breaths to regain control. I thought

## Chapter 1 – Conquering 'I Can't'

of the words Julie said: 'There's no such thing as can't.'

I was surprised at my ability to balance, still holding my position on the grey mat. I waited in fear to see if Julie was going to come and breathe fire on me.

She entered the small room again. 'Have you calmed down, Donna?' When I nodded determinedly to let her know I was brave, she knelt down beside me and said in her normal calm voice, 'Donna, I can put you back in your wheelchair or you can give this a go. You stayed up by yourself then, well done!' She was back to the nice Julie I knew all along; maybe she was having a bad day before.

But she was right, I did stay up by myself! Feeling pleased with myself, I decided to try crawling.

This was not easy. It was a struggle for my strange wonky body to balance, and for my mind to stay focused on the task and not give up. Julie was there to support me, to help me get back on my feet.

Little did I realise at the time, she had given me the power to make an important choice. To either go back as a victim in a wheelchair or become a person who wanted to get back on my feet, literally and mentally speaking. Hence the quote I use a lot now: 'The power is in me!'

I made that choice back then because I wanted to be able to play with my brother and sisters again, and I wanted to go back to school and play with my friends. Other reasons included what I *didn't* want. I didn't want people looking down at me in my wheelchair with a look of sympathy and pity. This was not the girl I wanted to be known as, and I did not want to be a hassle to my parents and family.

Julie had given me a massive lesson that day, to remember for the rest of my life: 'There's no such thing as can't.' This has stayed in my memory forever and I thank Julie for the lesson that truly made an impact on my life.

Occupational therapy was an everyday event that I attended after being able to get out of bed, similar to my visits to the physio department. This involved working to improve on my 'claw-like' hand that had lost the movement and capabilities I'd once had as a right handed child. This was a major task and I needed to show patience, endurance and determination.

There were plenty of fun activities such as cooking, art, painting, etc. to keep us interested and entertained. The simple act of mixing a bowl of cake mixture with my right hand and arm was considered a great achievement. Using a paintbrush to slop giant unrecognisable brush strokes on a piece of paper was a cause of further encouragement from the OT staff.

The more difficult, painful and frustrating moments in OT usually involved fine motor skill tasks, such as picking up pegs from an ice-cream container and placing them in another container. The space between the containers grew wider and more challenging over time, with the pegs and containers shrinking in size.

There have been hurdles in my life, but also so many great moments and outcomes from the results of these challenges. The people I have met. The challenges that push me to do things that I may not have otherwise tried.

We all have those moments of where we question our belief in ourselves, and our capabilities.

There's no such thing as can't. What a magical statement! They are words that can still be argued with, I'm sure. The statement to me is about trying, giving it a go, finding another way, finding a solution and asking the question, 'How can I?'

*'It's the things you fight for and struggle with before earning that have the greatest worth. When something's difficult to come by, you'll do that much more to make sure it's even harder – or impossible – to lose.'*
– Sarah Dessen

There are times where things seem so difficult and impossible to do. But when we really want to do it, why let limiting beliefs get in the way? There is a way, if we think about it more! We just need to open up to the idea of possibilities, where we may even have to ask for help.

Asking for help is not giving up or showing a weakness, as people think. Asking for help is opening up doors to other options or opportunities that you hadn't even thought about at the time, on your own.

A fresh approach can offer help, a chance to view the issue as a challenge with a solution from an angle that we haven't yet seen or thought about.

So asking for help is smart and resourceful. It is a solution to help you get positive results against the word and idea of 'can't'.

Those words I will never forget: 'There's no such thing as can't.' They were tough words to hear as an eight year old, but I am so glad Julie said them. I've reflected on that statement often, when I have been through tough times. So yes, I have had a few hurdles to jump over in my life, but these words have made me stronger.

Initially when you face a challenge, you need to decide, 'Can I? *How* can I?' But the thing is, after conquering 'I can't', you need to maintain focus.

Believing you can is the most important step of all. Remember, it's okay to ask for help or even stumble. Pick yourself up and do not be too proud to ask for help – people are always willing. And I find when people ask me now for advice and help, physically or mentally, I really love helping people – that's why I'm writing this book.

And you'll find also, whatever goal you have, if you approach the 'go-to person' – the person who's already done it, who's experienced this same challenge, who you look up to – they generally love getting that acknowledgement. To start with, you are interested in what they're doing, what they've done and how they've inspired you. They also just think, *Hey, this person's cool, I love that they've got this challenge, of course I want to help.*

So please, accept help when you see it, but also go out and seek it. Seek help if you find that you've got a block; this is not the time to stop.

*Chapter 1 – Conquering 'I Can't'*

Making the decision can be the scariest thing, as you'll see in the next chapter, but like with my big scary marathon, once I made the decision, that's when things happened. So I really advise you to focus on what you can do to reach your big scary goal (or goals). This is where you focus on each baby step that I'll lead you through in the book. You'll see how to do this for yourself, which is really exciting, because that's what this is about: for you to achieve your own big goal.

In the story with Julie, my big goal was to walk; this was where I focused on each baby step. The crawling, for instance, was one step toward my walking goal. Then after that, there was being able to kneel; after that, being able to stand … and so on.

These steps lead you closer to your big goal. This is why I really believe in the Baby Step Method to focus on the next baby step, rather than always focusing on the huge, big goal that looks really scary and too far away to reach. It's easy to give up when something gets in the way of the 'big goal' and it seems a little bit too hard – then this can become a habit, which in the long run doesn't get you anywhere.

I advise you to focus on each baby step, one at a time, but still having a clear picture of your end goal. It's important to have your mind set on that final goal, but focus on one step at a time – this will get you to your big goal, to your finish line.

# Chapter 2

# Choosing Your Distance

Having clarity in your personal or business life can sometimes be tricky to pinpoint. I will demonstrate here how you can get past the start line, with a clear path and an 'I can' attitude.

There are many benefits you'll get from this, but firstly it will remind you that this is your goal – it's nobody else's goal, you own it.

When you own it and have the clarity of what the goal is about, you gain certainty. You know when you're going to start this goal, and you know when you're going to end it. Make a statement that's specific about your goal and an end date. This gives you the certainty and confidence to move forward, which then gives you courage. Have you ever noticed that before?

Knowing what you want at a deeper, emotional level is always right – trust it. I always say, go with your gut feeling.

What will happen if you don't get to choose your own goal? You'll get stuck. You'll move in a direction that doesn't really benefit you, in your personal life, at work or even in business, and then you'll just lose direction.

This is where people just stop at the *idea* of their goal and it doesn't actually happen. And I don't want this to happen to you! This chapter is about clarity: a clear direction of where and how you can move to get your big goal.

So how do you regain certainty? Well, you create a plan; that's why I follow the Baby Step Method that you'll find later on in this book. It's what I've used for my big goals. I've also helped other people with their goals and this is how they've achieved it, using the Baby Step Method.

I encourage you to use this method and set a date. I hear you saying, 'I've set dates before and I've failed.' Make it realistic. I've mucked up with timing and dates as well, when I thought I could do something quicker. I'm the type of person who likes something done yesterday. Like this book, for instance; I would have liked it to be out in a certain time that I chose, but then I spoke realistically to the publisher and they gave me a reasonable bracket of time. Then I set a date in that bracket of time.

For the marathon, it was easy to choose the date, because that was already an organised event. It was 13 October 2013.

That time was made for me. Initially I thought eleven months wasn't going to be enough time for me to train to get over the finish line. But I got advice from my coaches Shaun and Chris, who said 'Yes, this is doable.'

So it's always good to get advice, like I did with my publisher and with my coaches. Get the advice from the experts and then make that date, because sometimes we can pull the time out of nowhere and it's just not going to happen because the date isn't realistic. Sometimes we just say, 'Oh yeah, someday I'll do that,' and that 'someday' never happens.

I need to emphasise the importance of making a plan – draw it up, type it up, whatever works for you. Put it somewhere where you see it every day; for instance, when I did the marathon training, I had a plan set up and I even said to Shaun, 'You can tell me to do things on certain days, but I'm actually a visual person and need it structured.' As a result, he wrote down exactly what I needed to do, including times and effort. I knew what I to do every day of the week and I put it in a Baby Step Method format for me to follow every day.

That's what worked for me! You may like pictures. Some people I know have vision boards with pictures of the things that they want and the things that they're aiming for. But as always, make sure there's a plan in place for you to get what's on your vision board.

I stuck my Baby Step Method plan on the outside of my wardrobe door. The plan changed and it grew, and that's what the baby steps are about. The baby steps are about starting small and increasing the intensity because you're improving and getting closer to your goal.

It's very exciting. So write a plan, put it somewhere you see every day and follow it.

I personally work with one big goal at a time, and advise that you do the same. This is what helps give me results to achieve. I'm not a multitasker when it comes to my big goals; from my experience this is where I failed and see others fail – let go of many goals at once!

Here's where I gained certainty with my marathon goal. It took a little time to decide, but like most big goals, it was initially a little scary.

### #training #lesson
### November 2012 – Learning about certainty

Emails went back and forth among Shaun, Chris and me, trying to work out a time when we could all meet in person. It was obvious that we all led busy lives, so to connect in the same place in the flesh at the one time seemed quite a challenge, even before the marathon challenge.

Chris was unable to make a time to catch up with us and said he trusted Shaun to handle the meeting with me and deliver their proposal – or was it me delivering a proposal? I so desperately wanted Chris there; I was depending on him for sanity in their partnership.

On 22 November, the day came when I was to meet Shaun for the first time in the flesh. I had many thoughts whirling in my mind, mostly from that day when my not-yet-confirmed coach made what seemed like a crazy suggestion.

I stepped into the café looking suspicious, like I was on a blind date. But I had seen a black and white photo of Shaun on his website, wearing glasses and looking very respectable and intelligent. Even though I knew this man was intelligent by the credentials listed on his website, it clearly hadn't stopped him from being a little crazy either if he still believed in his marathon idea.

The café was completely empty, making it easy for me to realise he was running late and that this wasn't a very popular café. A man entered catching my attention immediately – I looked but it wasn't him.

I turned away to see the person behind the counter smile at me as I kept looking out the window and toward the door, feeling like I was about to sit a verbal exam. The cold, sparse café gave no comfort.

Another man walked in, looking around. He saw me, smiled, and walked confidently toward me. He had spectacles, dark hair and a calm manner. It was definitely Shaun. Well, he appeared reasonably sane. I stood up, shook his hand and we began our relay of a serious conversation. He expressed how he could help, and I responded with my hope of fundraising for a cause I held close to my heart, as well as encouraging people that there's no such thing as can't.

My initial observation when this madman sat down was how big his eyes were and how they seemed to hold my attention. Were they just big from his magnified spectacles? Or was it from his very intense look and how he spoke about his passions, as well as his keenness in listening to mine?

Shooting back and forth like a game of tennis, I think it was obvious how passionate we both were about our aspirations. That was one thing we had in common.

We spoke about his suggestion of the marathon again, with me voicing my initial concerns of going backwards, maybe causing injury from all the work I had put into my body, from the stroke to where I am today. No decision was made at that point.

Parting in the street and turning to walk away, I wondered if this stranger was watching me walk with my usual hobble, thinking to himself, *What the hell have I just done?*

He could have been watching me walk along the busy city street, seeing the effort I need to put in to walk, especially in the shoes I wore with a slight heel. This would not be impressing my 'could-be coach' as I wasn't wearing the leg brace that lifts my toes, which helps me with my 'foot drop' – but the brace base did not fit in these slender, more dressy shoes.

It takes more effort to walk and lift my right foot so I don't trip on my toes, hence the foot drop that doesn't allow my toes to raise when walking. This sounds very complicated to the average person, but it has become a part of my life.

So I tried to walk as best as I could, without him noticing the effort I needed to put in. Why was I even doing this? Who was I trying to convince, Shaun or me?

I was not feeling confident in this challenge that started from an idea of running thirty steps to a 4 km fun run, which now turned into 42.2 km. How did I even get to this moment, this conversation, and this scary proposal?

I hopped on a tram and sat to contemplate this proposal on my journey home. I checked my phone to see a quote on Facebook that appeared straight away in my news feed – this was for me! Words that dissolved my 'what ifs' into insignificance; words that changed my thinking in that moment of contemplation:

*Chapter 2 – Choosing Your Distance*

*'I've missed more than 9000 shots in my career. I've lost almost 300 games. Twenty-six times, I've been trusted to take the game winning shot and missed. I've failed over and over and over again in my life. And that is why I succeed.'*

The quote was from legendary basketballer Michael Jordan.

That same day, I received an email from Shaun:

*Hey Donna,*

*It was great to spend some time with you this afternoon getting to know your story.*

*Clearly you have some reservations about what I'm suggesting for you, and your ability to carry it out.*

*Now, I don't know you very well at all, but from what you've told me about your life, it seems that you have already discovered that anything is possible with enough determination. What I'm offering you is guidance, knowledge and encouragement. What I ask in return is faith in Chris and me and a commitment to do whatever it takes to get the job done.*

*I would never endanger your health and you will have the option to pull out at any stage (but keep in mind that the pain of regret is far worse than the pain of failure).*

*You have an amazing story and the best part is that it is still evolving, and now you have the opportunity to do something that will make a big noise and help so many people in so many ways (both through the fundraising and through being an inspiration).*

*I'm going to make the decision about the marathon very easy for you. There are two options:*

*1) You can decide that a marathon is just nuts and we can call it off.*

*2) You agree to the marathon and Chris and I will hold your hand through the whole thing, helping with the training, publicity, the lot.*

*I know I'm being pushy here, and that is generally not my nature, but I feel very strongly about you doing this and KNOW that you can.*

*To put the pressure on even more, I'm giving you until 8 am tomorrow to tell me that you are going to take option 1 or option 2. Either way, the decision has to be yours and it has to feel right to you. Fear is okay; in fact, unless you are afraid of your goals, they aren't big enough.*

*I look forward to hearing from you.*

*Shaun.*

An ultimatum? I had less than twenty-four hours to get back to him with a decision to play or walk away. This guy was not just a pretty face; he was also clever and sneaky!

What shone past this guy's intensity and enthusiasm was his confidence in being able to help me with my challenge, even though he hadn't done any physical examination. I'll admit I was wary of this initially, trying to look at this objectively.

I'll admit, it took longer than the 8 am cut off decision time. This was a huge scary goal for me! It's sometimes tough to make that commitment. I'll talk more about the power of commitment in chapter 4.

I was still in two minds. I did think a marathon was nuts, but I also wanted Chris and Shaun's help, and I do like a challenge – 'I will try anything once,' I explained in an SMS to Shaun the next morning, after many SMS messages before.

Shaun's response: *Donna, 'Do or do not, there is no try'*, quoting Yoda. (I had no idea who Yoda was at that time).

The decision was made then, thanks to Yoda.

I decided I was learning to run again with Shaun and Chris. My big scary goal was to run the Melbourne Marathon on 13 October 2013. I had gained certainty, set a date, and I had eleven months to train. My next step was to make a plan, and that's what I did with these two crazy but awesome coaches.

His words from our initial phone conversation kept echoing in my mind: 'Donna, anyone can run a marathon – it's all to do with your mindset.'

I kept those golden words in my mind, all the way through this scary big goal. I encourage you to find your motivational quote to get you to your finish line.

# Chapter 3

# Finding Your Core

Identifying your reasons *why* drives you to keep your focus. Your emotions behind your desire are very important to reach your big scary goal. Why is your goal important to you?

In this chapter you'll also find out how discovering that *why* will give you clarity from what I was talking about in the previous chapters, and how important it is to have clarity on your big, scary goal.

The *why* helps not just yourself, but also other people around you. The *why* will keep you on track. When I was training for the marathon, at times I asked myself, 'Why am I doing this?' When it came to hard days, when I was struggling on my own, I did ask myself why. It brought me back to my reasons why – and I thought in that moment, 'I'm going to keep going.'

People ask me all the time, 'Donna, how do you keep yourself motivated?' It always comes back to my *why*. Your personal history also can be connected to your *why* – that's exactly what happened to me.

I didn't just have one *why* for my marathon goal; I had a number of whys. It was great having more than one, because it kept me thinking about all the reasons why I was doing it. This helped me to never give up.

What will you find when you drill down and keep asking yourself *why, why, why*? This is when it gets deeper and more emotional. This keeps you going through your baby steps, even when it gets really tough.

What I call 'drilling down' is illustrated in Terry's story, for example: he's a person who wanted to try to stop smoking. When I heard the word 'try,' it wasn't strong enough for me, so I asked, 'Will you try or are you going to actually do it?' My next question to Terry was, 'Why do you want to give up smoking?'

His first answer was, 'Because my kids tell me I stink.'

I asked again: 'Is there any other reason why?'

He said, 'Yeah, because I'd like to be more fit and active, and I don't feel like I can be when I smoke. I don't … my breathing, I have complications with that and I want to be able to play with my children.'

I thought that was a good reason. 'Is there anything else? What purpose will it give you? Is there any other reason why?'

He said, 'Well, I think my wife would prefer it if I didn't smoke either.'

I thought, *Here we go, this is getting deeper, he's thinking about other people,* but I wondered if there was anything

*Chapter 3 – Finding Your Core*

for himself in this as well. We kept going and it came down to Terry wanting to be around for his kids when they were grown up. 'I want to be able to walk my daughter down the aisle when she gets married.' This was a deep reason and I could see it in his eyes as they started to well up at that deep emotional level of that thought – that this may not happen if he keeps smoking.

For Terry, his *why* was so strong, once he really thought about it and said it aloud. He mentioned many important things to him. His children, his wife – these are all important people. But when it comes down to your own emotional *why*, something that really touches your heart, you're going to keep going and not give up on your goal. It's going to keep you on track.

It was hard at times for me. Completing a marathon by October 2013 was a huge goal; it was more obvious at times when I was struggling and I could only walk instead of run anymore in a training session. Whether you are a runner or not, you may understand that there's times when you really do lose energy, when you only have so much puff left, but I wanted to keep moving forward; I didn't want to stop.

You want to know my reasons, my *why*? Firstly, I was doing this as a personal challenge; it was a big challenge for me, and exciting.

Then there was also raising funds for the Royal Children's Hospital. That was a big reason to keep going, because I both made this promise to myself, and made a commitment to the hospital that I would support, in any way I could, the hospital that's helped so many children (including myself).

I had also told so many people; I started a Facebook page, and then a website. I had (and still have) an enthusiastic and encouraging following – I absolutely enjoy the people there, and I keep encouraging them to follow their dreams.

I did a lot of interviews with newspapers, magazines and radio programs. I told a lot of people, and felt that they were the reason why I kept going. I had made this promise and commitment and just thought, *I don't really want to go back on my word, I'm not that sort of person.* That was a big reason why as well.

My family had been a great support to me throughout my life – my parents especially, who are very strong people, but also my brother Brian; he was a very strong reason for me to keep going.

I was doing this for the seven year old Donna too. This may sound strange, but I had this image in my mind of my young enthusiastic self at seven, cheering me on from the side of the track when I trained on those tough days.

You may say to yourself, 'I don't have anyone to "drill down" with me, like with Terry.' Do it with yourself! I did. Or write it down on a piece of paper, getting right down to the deep *why*. When you do that, you'll find that you're open and honest about it. Ask yourself, 'What purpose will this give me?'

You can just stop at one *why*, but if you want to get deeper, go ahead: be brave and keep asking yourself. That's what I did with Terry, once we got down to the purpose that it would give him. It's worked with a variety of goals: weight loss, business, running goals, etc.

I had someone recently just say to me, 'It's something that I've always wanted to do, but you know, I don't think I'm good enough.' Find the reasons why you want to do it and you *make* yourself good enough. I find this keeps you on track when things really get hard.

But there's other things you can do to keep on track, like

keep pictures of your reasons why as constant reminders. It could be a family photo or a picture of a new house. If it's a travel goal then it could be a photo of where you want to go. You have to do something to get to that reason why, right? Have a picture of that destination, whatever it is.

This is what I mentioned about my followers, the people in my life and my family. My picture in my mind of my end goal was of me running into the Melbourne Cricket Ground, which is a pretty big deal; that's a big stadium. I would run in, and I would have my friends and family and other people close to me there, waiting and cheering me. This image really kept me going.

But while I had that image, I did still ask, 'Why am I doing this?' even if I was heading for a smaller goal; for example, my first small baby step was a 5.3 km fun run. I wanted to get to that, but I was always looking further ahead and focusing on the image of the *big* goal – of what I imagined it would look and feel like. Who was I going to see? What was I going to see? What was I going to smell? I even had this idea I'd probably have tears when I run into the oval.

But the reality in the end was that I had this huge smile on my face and everyone else around me was crying, which was kind of uncanny.

Still, I had a picture or image that may not be exactly the same in the end, but it still gets you to your big goal. Have that picture that excites you – that's what keeps you going.

I want to reiterate: always remind yourself *why*. Especially when you're questioning yourself; this is the time when you need to get back to the original reason why you want this big goal so bad. There will be times in your big goal when you'll be questioning yourself and thinking, 'I might just stop this, it's too hard, it's just probably never going to happen.'

If you have that mindset, it never will happen. You've got to keep strong, have the 'I can' attitude and just keep focused on the goal. You'll hear so many people who have achieved great things talk about their *why*.

### #training #lesson
### December 2012 – Mindset focus

Brian's path was a strong example of finding my deep emotional reason for reaching my goal. It was the first time I practised this with my running challenge training. This was in my early days of training, even before having my first session with Shaun and Chris.

I stared at the other end of a path not far from my regular training track. The length of this path was only 0.09 km (yes I measured it), but to run from one end to the other without stopping was a huge challenge for me at the time. I wanted to test the mindset theory, the power that I knew was capable of anything, in order to run to the end of this challenging path without stopping.

I took a deep breath, as I often forgot to breathe while running. I made an arbitrary decision that I was running to the end of this path to save Brian's life; to save my brother from the growth that invaded his body. I wanted to see my brother clear of cancer and decided at that moment that I would do anything to rid it, even run nonstop to the end of this path as a gesture.

I ran, focusing my eyes on one spot; if anything got in my way I'm certain I would have ran over it. It was not about me being a hero at the end of the path and everyone cheering me. It was about my desperate plea to keep Brian alive to share his love, kindness, enthusiasm and loyalty to his wife, son, family, friends and even strangers that he would meet and connect with. To see him finally happy and excited as a husband and father was a joy for us all.

I made it to the end of the path that day. Telling you this still makes my eyes well up with tears, as that run, or any other run I did, didn't save Brian's life. However, even after our sad loss I was not about to stop. I will always remember his excitement, encouragement and enthusiasm when I first announced my marathon goal to him and my mission to raise funds for the RCH.

That path is a special place that I still go to now, where I have a place to sit in a beautiful garden, to reminisce about the time I had with Brian when he was alive and the good times we shared, and the impact he had on my life, and so many others.

*'I assess the power of a will by how much resistance, pain, torture it endures and knows how to turn to its advantage.'*
  – Friedrich Nietzsche

## Chapter 4

# Commitment Gives Power

We can all relate to the excitement of setting a big goal, and as time progresses it is only commitment that will give us the motivation and power to help us cross the finish line. Commitment will give you the 'never give up' attitude and it builds belief in yourself.

Commitment also inspires others, and is transferable to other areas in your life, not just this one big scary goal that you want to achieve right now. You can move it into other areas of your life, which is pretty exciting.

If you don't have that commitment, you would just stay stagnant. You'd be disappointed time and time again; disappointment in yourself sneaks up in other areas of your life, and doesn't do positive things for you mentally.

Commitment gives power. It's a great strategy for keeping motivation to reach a big goal. It's a strategy that works, especially when making that commitment to someone else.

Have you ever noticed that once you tell someone something, they always come back to you and say, 'Hey Joe, how's that project going?' You're committed now, because you've said it out loud. I don't know about you, but I feel that way.

> *'I am a success today because I had a friend who believed in me and I didn't have the heart to let him down.'*
> – Abraham Lincoln

This is accountability. When someone says, 'I don't know if I can do this or make that commitment,' I encourage them to get a coach or a mentor, or even use their buddies.

Buddies are probably the ones that you see more of in your day to day life, and if they keep asking you, 'How's that project going?' you're pretty much accountable to them.

You may think a coach would be a great accountability buddy, but say your response is, 'I can't afford to hire a coach.' Perhaps you can offer something in return, like a win-win situation – a business referral, perhaps. Remember, ask yourself, 'How can I afford a coach?' Work out a payment plan. This is what I do with my clients, if needed, so it is doable for them.

The option I chose, once I wanted to run again, was my coaches Shaun and Chris. I really felt I needed to have someone teach me to run again; I hadn't run in thirty-four years and I struggled to run thirty steps, so the first thing I thought was that I needed help. When I found Chris and Shaun and heard what they did as experts in running, I really wanted to have these guys on board, but I couldn't afford to have a coach at the time.

So we made an agreement: I helped them with promoting their business and they supported me in getting me up and running (literally!). So there's always a way.

I could have asked myself 'Can I afford a coach?' and I could have said no and just left it at that. But when you ask, 'How can I afford a coach?' you work out ways, don't you?

> *'When confronted with a challenge, the committed heart will search for a solution. The undecided heart searches for an escape.'*
> – Andy Andrews

But saying it out loud is a big thing – it kept me committed, that's for sure! I did it by creating social media profiles. I did it with friends, family and media. If you really want to be accountable and make that commitment, do all of these things and get to it.

Yet, saying it aloud can be terrifying.

On 23 November 2012, after attending a friend's art exhibition opening that evening, four of us went to have celebratory drinks afterwards. We got talking about our new year's resolutions for 2013.

When it came around to my turn, I tried to sound confident but I was initially frightened and trying not to reveal my crazy nervousness to them. I announced, 'I'm going to run a marathon in 2013.'

I did it! I'd said it out loud to a new group of people who looked at me with a mixture of reactions. Excitement, amazement or disbelief came from some, one even adding a humorous reaction to this.

This was scary, but at the same time, it was a relief just announcing it to these friends, like allowing oneself to breathe after receiving good news rather than bad, even though not everyone responded with a positive reaction.

However, I felt that I was ready to tell the world now, as I was able to unlock that slight apprehension of, 'What will people say? What if I fail?'

This is a big thing that many of us need to get over, worrying about what other people would say. But I knew it didn't matter at that moment; I was okay with it now. Yes, it is scary to put your big goal out there, but it's exciting too. I thought to myself, *I'm going to have all sorts of reactions so I may as well suck it up*.

Then with help from a friend, we created the Facebook page. I was a newbie at Facebook, so there we go again – asking for help from friends, the experts or whomever. It is okay to ask for help. I had no idea how to create an actual page or what to do with it. But this was where my major following began, which I am truly grateful for, to this day. You see, people who follow a FB page usually like it, right? So people were amazed with my challenge, but also very encouraging.

Another thing I think is important with commitment is keeping a journal, or recording daily or weekly accounts of your journey and your results: what works, what doesn't work, daily thoughts and so on, whatever you'd like to write.

Some people are more structured; some people like doing a journal, or as I call it, 'verbal vomit on a page'. It's good to do. My journal consisted of recording information to do with my diabetes. Chris asked me to keep a food diary and see what foods worked well with my day to day routine, including my running training sessions and diabetes monitoring. It was all a bit of a juggling act at first, and I'm naturally not keen on keeping a food diary, but this was a commitment I made.

I'd do more frequent blood tests, monitoring my BG (blood glucose) levels before I went out for a training session, then again when I came back, and found out what worked. Did my BG level go down or up? How was I feeling? I'd take sultanas or jelly beans with me, but working out the distance, and the time that I ran, did make a difference when I walked as to when I ran. I learned all this by recording the information – not just for myself, but to take it to my 'diabetes team': my diabetes educator, my dietician and my endocrinologist.

So it made me accountable in some ways, but also helped with other things I needed to do successfully. I believe in doing the journaling that is relevant to your goal. If you're not a big fan of writing, or find you don't have time, even record voice messages on your phone – whatever works for you! Then go back and listen to your recordings. You'll even hear with the sound of your voice sometimes how you sounded a bit uncertain – you can see how you've grown in confidence with what you're doing, how you're training and how you're getting to your goal. Then you may have some days when you feel like crap, and that's okay too; it's better to let it out than hold it in.

But it's always good to pick yourself up again. Like I always say, it's alright if you trip, stumble or have a crap day, but don't stay there too long – you can pick yourself up. It's how you respond to these stumbles is what gives you the results, so you choose.

Speaking of commitment, it's easy to make excuses too. We can all come up with excuses; we're such experts at it for some reason. There are times when it's difficult because of 'time', or maybe things are out of our control, such as weather.

I mention this to show you the focus that you can have, the things that you can alter or tweak to keep your commitment to your preparation and progress to your goal.

For example, with my marathon training sessions, there was a time where I was busy one week and I just couldn't run or even do a brisk walk at the usual times that I trained. One night it was dark and raining, but I thought, *I haven't done my walk today, I hadn't been active. I'm just going to go to the supermarket.*

So I was in my running gear, just pacing and speed-walking up and down the aisles at the supermarket. This sounds crazy, I know! I'm surprised I didn't have a security guard come and tap me on the shoulder. I just wanted to keep my focus and momentum on that commitment that I made. It isn't a hard thing to do, to commit and change things around – tweak or alter it if you have to, but make it happen.

There was also a week where I had four extended days of a training workshop for work, and I'm not an early morning person. But this particular week I still needed to keep active; I had to keep my commitment. That week I got up really early – it was still dark outside. I found I actually kind of enjoyed it, because it was so peaceful at the same time too.

Don't get me wrong, I didn't do mornings after that – I only did it for that week – but that's the sort of thing that you may have to change within your schedule to show flexibility. At the same time you're keeping your commitment – awesome!

> *'Most people fail, not because lack of desire, but because of lack of commitment.'*
>     – Vince Lombardi

## Chapter 5

# Jump Right Out

Moving out of our comfort zone is a major leap when going for your big goal, but this is where real action begins for us to reach that big goal.

Why? Well, it takes you to places you've never been to. It can be scary, but exciting too. When I'm facing a big challenge, people may ask, 'Are you scared, Donna?' And I've said at times, 'Well, yeah, it's a bit scary, but I'm excited too!'

That's what challenges are about. They help you to grow. And they're invigorating, too. So a good challenge will propel you to move forward, rather than backward when getting out of your comfort zone.

If you're doing something the same all the time and you're not getting anywhere with your goal, that's when you have to make a decision and say, 'What do I have to do differently?' Maybe you have to make that scary call you've been avoiding, or that conversation you've wanted to have with your boss to ask for that pay rise, or maybe you have to ... and so on. Or maybe you just have to say no for a change, instead of saying yes?

> *'If you want something you've never had, then you've got to do something you've never done.'*
> – Unknown

I find that when people do stay in their comfort zone, they get stuck or stay in the same spot. They're not reaching their goal, because they stay in fear of the unknown. They don't progress or move forward to reach their finish line. But we want you to reach the finish line; that's the reason why you're reading this book.

Science has found that a moderate level of uncertainty and anxiety can help people be ready for anything. People who are out of their comfort zones are better at multitasking and more aware of potential problems. Dr Stephen Josephson, a psychologist in New York City who has treated athletes, actors and musicians, states: 'Coaches and sports psychologists have always known that you don't want your athlete to be relaxed right before an event. You need some 'juice' to go fast.'

In the beginning, to move out of your comfort zone can be a huge, scary thing. When you make it a habit – to jump out and think outside the square to get to your goal – this is where the magic happens.

When it comes to moving out of your comfort zone, I also advise seeking a mentor: someone who's already done this particular goal, or something similar. You may not know anyone who has done what you want to do, and that can make it big and scary as well. But if you seek a mentor, that can be really helpful and get you charged.

Ask around. You may say, 'I don't know anyone to mentor me.' These are the times where you say it out loud. Perhaps you don't want to tell the whole world yet? Perhaps you just want to talk to close friends about it and ask them, 'Do you know anyone who has done this?' Maybe they'll be able to help you, or put the word out for you.

You need to do this! And it's going to be a challenge if you have to step out of your comfort zone. So I really encourage you to.

I have an exercise that I tell a lot of people to do, because it gets you into the habit of doing something different: do one scary thing every day. It can be smaller things, like making those calls that you need to do in your business, rather than something huge.

Make those ten sales calls that you've been putting on the bottom of your list every day, because you're making the excuse of needing to do this first, needing to do that first … but really, you know what you need to do. It's always on your list and you haven't done it yet because it's too scary.

Another scary thing that you could do is just say 'no' to someone. Are there things or people getting in the way of your goal because you always say 'yes' to everyone? Do you really like what you're saying yes to? Or are you saying yes because you find it difficult to say no? Are you a constant crowd pleaser who really isn't getting pleasure in your life, or getting closer to your goal finish line?

If you want to get to your goal on the date that you've set and move out of your comfort zone, you need to sometimes say no.

I needed to change what I knew of running and do things that were different and sometimes difficult for me. I was using muscles that I hadn't worked in thirty-four years.

I needed to follow my coach's directions, because he had done this before. He not only had helped other people who succeeded in their running goals, but he was someone who ran crazy ultra-marathons. I needed to trust that he would get me there and help me with my plan to complete a marathon.

Sometimes I hear people say, 'I can't change, I need to stay in my routine.' But really, has this helped them so far? Has that routine helped them get to this goal that they've found challenging, but always dreamed about?

Have you ever had such a big goal, something that you've dreamt about for so long? Now you can by taking action to change what you're currently doing, even by reading this book. It's one of the scary steps, getting out of your comfort zone, but it's a positive step.

> 'Move out of your comfort zone. You can only grow if you are willing to feel awkward and uncomfortable when you try something new.'
> – Brian Tracey

Be comfortable with getting out of your comfort zone.

Be open to change, to progress – this is how you will move forward.

*Chapter 5 – Jump Right Out*

## #training #lesson
## December 1978 – Breaking from the usual comfort

Most days at RCH had a basic routine: things like morning medication, breakfast, bed bath, bed change, cleaners going in and out. Groups of doctors came in everyday, right on cue like a herd of sheep, with their shepherd keeping them reared together, using big words I didn't really understand. Then I visited Julie, then OT, etc.

But this particular day was different. 'Donna, you're going for a visit!' claimed the Sister. She seemed very orderly, giving messages to two men who appeared by either side of my bed. One was wheeling another narrow funny rackety sounding bed with wheels, while the other man used his foot to adjust my bed with the lever to pump it up to the same height as their bed. I knew immediately what they were doing; I'd seen this before. They were moving me on the funny narrow bed. But why? Where were they taking me?

These men wore different uniforms from the rest of the team I was familiar with. 'We are going to take you on an ambulance ride, Donna. My name's Tony and this is David.'

David took a folder from the Sister, placed it at my feet at the end of the bed and smiled at me.

I was wheeled out of Ward 6 by the ambulance men. Mum wasn't there to come with me. Where were they taking me? The ambulance team spoke as if I should have been excited about a 'mystery tour'. 'We are taking you to the Royal Melbourne Hospital, Donna.'

My head turned and eyes searched all around as I raised my neck awkwardly, searching all around the room for my missing mum. Why wasn't she here? Did she know about this unexpected move? Did Mum know where to find me?

Why were they taking me to another hospital? Was there something wrong with this hospital?

Would I lose all contact with everyone who knew I was here? How could I let them all know?

Were they taking me to another room to prick my veins? Were they going to poke and torture my arms and tell me it will only be a small prick, like a mosquito bite, when it's not?

Were they lying to me? Was this a trick?

'Where's Mum?' My head swung from side to side, scanning the room.

'Donna, it is okay,' another voice told me in a calm manner, like it didn't matter that my mum wasn't with me. 'It is only a short visit. You will be back here this afternoon.'

I felt a little better from my anxious feeling of Mum not being with me, from knowing that I would be able to see my family and friends again in Ward 6. The ambulance men rolled me away on a bed with wheels, down the corridor of Ward 6, out into the elevator and through other parts of the building I found hard to recognise.

Looking up the noses of the ambulance men, I felt a breeze and saw flashes of movement buzz straight past me before I even had time to

*Chapter 5 – Jump Right Out*

see what I was actually passing. This brought a blurred flashback of the confusion from being in the ambulance in Mildura, going to the airport to fly to RCH.

Suddenly I felt cool air on my face; we must have been outside. But before I even got a moment to breathe in the fresh air, I was immediately in the cocoon. 'We're now in the ambulance to take you to the Royal Melbourne Hospital,' Tony said in his calm voice.

From one hospital to another; this didn't make sense.

'We are taking you to an appointment where there's a special machine that will do some tests on your head, Donna.'

*What's he talking about? My head is fine,* I thought to myself. Mum always came with me to new appointments. She always held my hand and made me feel safe. Mum knew everything and always explained to me what was happening.

How was I going to explain this to Mum? I barely understood what they said half the time. Mum knew what they said; she always explained things and asked just the right questions! What was I going to tell her?

Was Mum going to be alright on her own in Ward 6, when she got there to find my empty bed? What would she do on her own? Who would play Chinese checkers with her? What about our card game, and the book she was reading me? Will anyone explain to her where I've gone? Will she come to find me? Will she know where to find me?

The ambulance stopped. The two doors opened and I knew it was time to push me out and wheel me into the unknown. Into a noisy building and out into what seemed like a secret corridor, the rattly bed was on the move again. There was no use looking for Mum here; all I could do was look up Tony's nose and hope that he would take care of me.

We entered a silent room, where I heard a lady's soft voice. 'Mum?' I said hopefully.

'No,' Tony replied with a smile, 'this is a kind lady who will look after you here, Donna.'

Tony and David moved me from my bed with wheels onto another, more narrow hard bed that felt cold, topped with a stiff white sheet. Was this a bed or a metal plank? I think it was even more uncomfortable than seeing Dr Edmond the heart doctor, with the cold jelly and funny stick he used to poke around my chest.

At the head of the cold bed was a huge white shiny cave, like in a spaceship movie. It was very cold and not very inviting; this was scary. *What are they going to do now? Is this the cave that sucks me up into a dungeon, never to be found again? Will I see another human again?*

The big noisy cave slowly sucked me in, with my stiff scared body on the cold, hard plank with the hard white funny smelling cardboard sheet.

The ambulance men had left me here with two blue-gowned strangers wearing odd goggles. Feeling strange and scared of my new surroundings, one of the goggled blue strangers walked toward me. She looked down and put a surprisingly warm human hand on mine. 'It's okay, Donna, you're going to be fine. Try to be a brave girl. We will just be in the next room,' the lady's voice said.

As she walked away from me, my thoughts became more curious. *Brave for what?* I thought. *The noisy cave dungeon I was just about to enter?* I had heard those words before: 'Be a brave girl, Donna.' It usually ended up hurting.

A loud voice came from nowhere, making my fearful body jump. 'Donna, you have to lie very still for me. When you hear me say "now", that is when you must not move.'

Geez! How am I supposed to stay still when I have this loud voice coming from nowhere, telling me not to move and sounding very serious? Was this God or the Devil talking to me? Maybe it was the voice leading me to the dungeon? But it didn't sound like it was coming from the dungeon.

Why wasn't I allowed to move? Did I have to keep still for any reason? Why wouldn't anybody explain? Maybe I had to stay still to enter a crocodile's gigantic mouth that was waiting wide open at the other side of the cave!

At that moment I felt the bed bump and I was certain it must have been from the crocodile's breath!

With all these thoughts in my confused mind, I could no longer hold my anxious tears back. My frail body was shaking from my deep sobs, trying to catch each breath in between. I was trying so hard to be brave, but had little control over my panicked breaths and sobs. *Will I ever see Mum again, or Dad and my brother and sisters?*

The blue-gowned goggled person appeared before me, making me jump with fright. Taking her goggles away, she revealed long eyelashes, and eyes filled with concern and tolerance. 'Donna, this isn't going to hurt. We just need you to keep still for a few seconds each time, so that John can take photos of your head.'

'Is John the voice?' I thought out loud.

She nodded, pointing to the top of the spaceship cave that was taking me to the dungeon. 'That's what this big thing is for, to take photos like a giant camera. We need to be in the other room to do this. It won't take long if you try to keep as still as you can. Then I will come back in to see you,' she explained.

'Where is my mum?' I asked.

'I am sure she will be at RCH when you get back there,' the lady explained. 'My name is Sarah and I will take care of you today.' Sarah's voice was firm but calm. 'Now show us how brave you are, Donna.'

I was often asked to be brave at RCH; surely I could do it again here. I must be brave for Mum. She was always brave for me. I hoped she was okay in Ward 6, all alone without me. I had to be still for the gigantic camera so I could get back to Mum.

*Chapter 5 – Jump Right Out*

An unnerving feeling of loss of control and the unexpected or 'out of routine' situations are there to test us. I think my mum and dad would have had more than one of these experiences themselves, facing the unexpected and having no sense of control of the situations they faced at that time – and in the months and years ahead. But it is important how you deal with that sense of no control. I've always seen my parents as a great example of strength, adaptability and courage to move forward in a positive direction.

Feeling as though I didn't have my mum to be there as my comforter and support person was a big thing for me, as Mum was always there; she was my reason for living, she was my *why*...my family was my *why*.

But I had to be brave, to move forward in the challenge I faced, to get me on the road to improve my situation and reach my goal to get where I am today. I could not let her down. But I'm sure I have, more than once, when I think about it.

My parents showed so much courage in this difficult period. For many years after, they were tested, stretched and taken out of their comfort zone many times throughout this journey. In the end it was for a successful outcome.

Yes, I did survive the Royal Melbourne Hospital visit. Now I see it as overreacting, but that can come from being in a situation of the 'unknown' or being out of your comfort zone, even for the most courageous people. We can over-analyse and create ridiculous thoughts in our mind, even to the point of thinking they are real excuses that stop us from moving out and closer to our goal ... because we start believing the excuses are a true reason not to go for our goal. Even though they sound crazy ... like a crocodile!

> *'Always go a little further into the water that you feel you're capable of being in. Go a little bit out of your depth. And if you don't feel your feet are about to touch the bottom, you're just about in the right place to do something exciting.'*
> – David Bowie.

## Chapter 6

# Training Buddies

Who are you hanging out with? Are you surrounding yourself with buddies who are encouraging, supportive or maybe even experienced in the goal you want to achieve?

At different speaking events, even with students, I always speak about the importance of creating a positive support system when you really want to reach your big goal.

It's a great advantage, especially when you're supported by people who have already done it. But if you don't have that support system, be aware of who is in your network: that includes family, friends, even your colleagues. Are they the people who are really giving you support? Or are they the people putting you down and ignoring you when you want to talk about your challenge and your big goal, and show how excited you are?

Are the people who surround you and hang out with you an encouraging group? This is important, because behaviours can be contagious. I'll give you an example. Have you ever been to a friend's backyard barbecue party? You enter the backyard and there's a group in the corner; you join the conversation and listen to what they're saying, and one person is talking about how they had a really bad day that week, but they're okay now. But he continues to list all of the bad events for that day and how bad it was. Then everyone else joins in. They all say, 'Well, I've had that before too,' or, 'Oh yeah, I know exactly where you've been,' and list all their bad events/days they've had too. They go on and on, like it's a competition of who in the group has had the worst day ever! It's a contagious conversation. People talk about similar things, right?

So who are you hanging around with? Are they encouraging? And when you talk about your exciting project, are they excited for you? Make sure that you're excited for them as well; it's give-and-take, isn't it? That's what buddies are about. They keep you motivated and you do the same with others, because that's what you'll attract. Buddies can cheer you on and they can boost your confidence.

Remember, from confidence comes courage. This includes gaining confidence from positive feedback. But some people may not have this in their life and they're feeling alone. I've heard a lot of people, especially when they're in their own business as entrepreneurs, saying they just get down. They say, 'This is a lonely game.' Especially when they don't have many people in their business; they may be a one man/woman 'show', so to speak.

But then some might be hanging around the wrong company who's saying the same thing. They might be around other people who are in the same business and they are all saying the same negative talk that gets them down. With this so-called support, it can end up seeming like you're the only person in the world who has a big dream; it's easy to give up in that negative situation. We can easily take on other people's doubts or fears and bad advice – but we don't want that for you.

They say that you are what you eat. Have you heard that? What about, you are whom you hang around with? From what I've seen and experienced of behaviours, it seems that behaviours are contagious – whether positive or negative.

I experienced this with my adventure programs. People join my group adventure programs for a reason: they want to do something exciting that they haven't done before. Usually they haven't known how to get there, or a little bit of fear has held them back. But when you get with a likeminded group that is so excited about the adventure program challenge, they all have this excitement; keeping the motivation going in the group. We have tough times and we have times where we laugh and carry on, but we're doing it together with the same attitude and also encouraging each other. And with encouragement and support from me, they are learning, growing and stepping out of their comfort zone.

It becomes a contagious behaviour and that's what really moves you forward. It helps to keep you going.

With my marathon goal, I firstly created a following. What I did was extreme, probably, but I created a following for Run Donna Run with a Facebook page, Twitter and Instagram profiles and even a blog on my website. I created this following where people were interested and encouraging. People are only going to follow you if they like what you're doing, especially in social media. They may feel amazed with what you're doing and haven't done it before themselves, but like to watch and they encourage you – this is like having a massive team of training buddies who encourage you with their contagious positive behaviour.

But also connect with others who've done it. I did that with other people who had run marathons. You could say, 'I don't know anyone, it's hard to make friends in that area of my challenge, because there's nobody I know in my network, my friends don't do it.' Look it up on the internet; look up groups in your niche. There are Facebook groups or Meetup groups for everything. Or even create a group of your own – either network groups or social groups.

I really encourage getting out there, joining a social club, and catching up one on one with people who are aiming for a similar goal or have already done it. It's amazing, the people I've come in contact with who were interested in knowing what I was doing.

For example, I contacted people I held in high regard; they'd written books about their journey of running marathons and ultra-marathons. It's amazing the people you can contact through a private message in Facebook. I told them just a little bit about what I was doing and how excited I was. It's awesome the response I got from people. They were really interested and they did find the time to catch up – that was a boost to me! It's like having a training buddy in a way, because they're going to really boost and encourage you along the way. And be sure to check in with them; I'm so sure they'll respond to see where you're at and encourage you.

Finally, choose your friends wisely. And this is where people say to me, 'Well, I can't just dump my friends.' I'm not suggesting to dump friends, but maybe hang around them less often for a while, in favour of those encouraging you and supporting your goal.

People come in and out of our life for a reason. Spend less time with the negative and more time with the positive friends, if you find it hard to let go. I often say, especially if there's people who are really close to you (such as your partner or your family), to put them on mute, like with your TV remote control. But sometimes we just have to let it go. Some people put their own doubts and fears on you. But never own it; that's their issue, not yours.

*'You had a purpose before anyone had an opinion.'*
– Unknown

### #training #lesson
### 1978 – Contagious behaviours

Brian, Anne and Toni, my siblings, visited me with Dad for the first time at RCH. It was so good to see recognisable faces. I still had no speech, and lay in bed the whole time, but I was aware of what was happening and they were still able to play with me.

They played with a little figure of a man, with shiny bright coloured limbs that were connected with elastic. When Brian continuously pressed underneath the box the funny man was standing on, the smiling man changed into all sorts of positions. Bending back, to the side, then forward – and when released he stood straight again, like a soldier standing to attention.

This made us all laugh! It was great to see my family!

No matter how many times Brian, Anne and Toni all took turns to take control of this funny toy, we laughed and laughed like it was the first time we saw the crazy movements of the plastic man's body. It amused us for quite some time, but seeing my brother and sisters was the underlying happiness for me. It made a difference to be surrounded by my loved ones.

It's funny how sound can be made with laughter. There are no words to put together when laughing, but still it makes a pleasant, joyous sound that is contagious and unique to each individual. I am grateful for still being able to laugh even through tough times, even when I could not speak, thanks to the wonderful people around me.

*'Laughter is the best medicine!'*
– Unknown

Even to this day when I see that kind of toy, I relate it to the memory of being speechless in hospital and having my brother and sisters around me in laughter.

It's a great memory, knowing how sick I was and how the importance of my family being around me made me feel. Laughter is not silent and my family's presence is always felt within me, even when I am away from them.

Really, what I'm saying here is how important it is to focus on getting a training buddy (or buddies) – on finding that positive contagious behaviour and identifying encouraging people to surround yourself with.

Using the example of running again, I know many runners who like to run with a friend; this keeps them accountable. This also applies to working out at a gym, and having a goal

*Chapter 6 – Training Buddies*

to lose weight. Some people find it scary even to open the gym door, but if you find a supportive person to train with, this makes you accountable and makes the routine more enjoyable – and achievable.

Remember to make your journey fun!

## Chapter 7

# Mental Roadblocks

When thinking of our big goal, whether it's what we've wanted for a long time or something new we've been dreaming of, sometimes it's easy to make excuses as to why we can't achieve it. This is what I call a mental roadblock. But how about instead we find a solution as to how we can achieve your big goal?

As a benefit, you'll clear your mind of negative thoughts. When we can interpret this as a growth in ourselves, instead of fear of change or challenges that come our way, then this can turn them into opportunities. It's scary but it's exciting, and you may inspire others to achieve their dreams too.

Do you look at a mental roadblock as a challenge or a threat? I like to look at it as a challenge. Challenge is a more exciting word. But if you don't get past these mental blocks, you're just going to be stuck – and that may be where you are right now. Perhaps that's why you're reading this book. I really want to help you with this, so you don't fall into a hole and focus on what you can't do, but instead find out how you can and why you want to do it.

Challenges are difficult, yes. That's why it's called a challenge. Not everybody achieves them. People fall into the pattern of staying in their mental block.

Your goal is an amazing challenge that you *are* going to achieve. We will cover more of this in the next chapter.

I think a good piece of advice is to turn your struggle or roadblock into a success story. Your first baby step creates an impact for the mindset of the rest of your journey.

> *Alice: 'This is impossible!'*
> *Mad Hatter: 'Only if you believe it is.'*
>     – Lewis Carroll

For example, a 5.3 km run changed everything for me, and that was just my first baby step. Your first small goal creates a positive impact on your mind.

### #training #lesson
### January 2013 – My first running event

It was 5.45 am when my alarm woke me. After a disturbed sleep, I wasn't nervous. I had a low blood glucose level in the middle of night, but felt good with a BG reading of 8.7 when waking in the morning. I gave myself a little less insulin, with a wholesome breakfast to prepare for my very first ever fun run challenge.

*Chapter 7 – Mental Roadblocks*

I knew this wasn't a marathon, just 5.3 km, so I had what I would normally eat any other day; even though Chris was trying to get me off the muesli to eat fewer carbs, I wasn't sure of that yet. I tested my BG again after breakfast and it was 9.5; I was cool with that – diabetes can be challenging at times.

I was excited about this new challenge and feeling okay. A friend took me on the long drive to the Rosebud Australia Day Fun Run, grabbing my BG machine again before getting out of the car: 5.9, perfect! I had my sultanas with me as advised by Chris. This was a test for me, and a huge step in my eyes … my very first running event!

Start – go! Running along the road (and remembering to keep to the left as Shaun said), I stuck to my pace after the excitement of a rushed crowd was over. I slowed to a walk sooner than I would've liked, thinking, *Listen to your body, don't overdo it at the beginning.* Talking to myself in my mind was a common occurrence since beginning this new running challenge, often hearing Shaun's voice butt in as well.

At the halfway mark, I struggled at this stage to keep momentum and with a sore left shin, probably from overcompensating with my stronger side, I saw a man on the sideline ahead … was he waving to me? I looked around to see if anyone was responding to this tall man with a camera in hand pointing my way. I realised it was Chris as I got closer – *oh crap*, I thought, *he's filming me while I'm struggling*, but it was a buzz to see him!

I didn't think he would travel so far, as he didn't live close, to cheer me with his words of encouragement: 'Keep going, ruuun!' His enthusiasm picked me up as I refocused and ran off. I was so grateful for him being there that day, as this was a big challenge for me.

Meeting people along the way was also encouraging. I chatted with two kids at one stage who were curious about my leg brace; I explained my past in brief and how this was my first ever running event, and in return listened to their stories of the running events they'd already completed and others they were planning to achieve. They were fun and truly inspiring. What I love about children is their honesty, curiosity and enthusiasm.

Crossing the finish line was a huge moment for me; hearing my name mentioned before crossing the line was cool too. Receiving my first ever medal was awesome and getting the event show bag was great. I felt like an excited kid at a carnival.

Seeing my friend was a relief as I ran toward her with a huge smile, waving my medal with pride and relief. I was happy to see her familiar face among the crowd, with her camera in hand of course, excited and asking me questions while filming. She gave me a huge hug that I was truly grateful for. I then found Chris, and a couple of other supporters with him too. This is something I will never forget.

This always brings a huge smile to my face when telling this story. It was a huge achievement for me – and yes, I had a fixed smile on my face, ready for my next challenge.

A happy day: 5.3 km at 45.32 minutes. I of course wore my first ever medal for the rest of the day, even at a friend's Australia Day barbecue.

This 5.3 km run was the first major step out of my 'baby steps' to my goal, which I now preach about both at speaking events and to people who say, 'A marathon is huge!' or those who ask, 'How did you do it?'

This run was very significant in increasing my strength, both mentally and physically. Self-belief is very important when reaching for any goal; this is no different to any other goal that you may have, and it doesn't need to be running. This is my message that I wanted to share and spread: 'Believe you can ...'

After that was my next baby step: my goal was a 10 km run. After the 5.3 km run that I just completed, I said, 'I can do that, I just have to double what I just did today!'

What I enjoyed about this run was the fact that people who ran beside me or even past me were encouraging each other, and that is something I really love to see.

I prefer to train alone, so to be in an environment surrounded by thousands of runners who were of varied ages and abilities, male and female, all in it for different reasons, was an awesome feeling. But aside from completing the distance, gaining confidence in my ability to keep going was my result in this particular run.

The response I had from people who followed me on my Facebook page was awesome. I was truly grateful to those who followed and cheered me on, including my family and friends ... who may or may not have believed in me initially.

My friend kept people posted on my Facebook page and sent photos. So when travelling home from the run I was flabbergasted to see an endless amount of messages on my phone and on my Facebook page.

Then there was a reaction from a less encouraging friend: 'You know Donna, even if you just do the 10 km run everyone will be impressed. If you don't make the full marathon, don't worry about it.'

Although this friend may have thought of this comment as encouraging, this thought never entered my mind. Maybe this was his concern, or his own fear, when I announced my next step of completing a 10 km run. That night I decided that I wouldn't hang out with that friend 'as much' throughout my training, and surrounded myself with positive people. This was very important to me at that stage and this made me think of Brian.

I knew that was what he wanted from people around him: to be positive and not get him down with negative talk while fighting the cancer. This I could do for him – if I had no other power to control his situation, I knew I could be a positive energy around him, for him.

> 'Surround yourself with people that reflect who you want to be and how you want to feel, energies are contagious.'
> – Unknown

I was grateful for my followers on my Facebook page. These were people who only knew me for a month on Facebook, but they inspired me every day. This was a blessing that helped me to keep on track. Although I continued thanking them,

*Chapter 7 – Mental Roadblocks*

I wondered if they realised how important their response to my marathon goal was to me. They were awesome!

I look at this first 5.3 km running challenge as something almost bigger than the actual marathon, funnily enough, because I shifted so much in my mindset to complete this first baby step goal, which took away the mental roadblock that I may initially have had.

But you may think, 'I'm not a success story.' You will be though, especially in the eyes of others who may want to achieve the same goal. That's when you become a success story; that's when you become an example to people of how it can be achieved. It's exciting!

Remember: whenever you say 'I can't' in your head, instead ask yourself, 'How can I? Why am I doing this?' This will clear your roadblocks, I'm certain.

Another important way to get over the roadblocks is to keep in mind how you want to achieve the goal and what the big picture will look like: the feelings, the smells or even tastes that will go with it. Get clear on the vision to the end, even through the tough times.

I remember doing this when I was training, with my vision of entering the MCG. I held that close to me: that thought, that vision. I'd close my eyes, seeing it happen, seeing the people who were there, the feelings and the sounds of people cheering – and of me feeling proud. That's what was always in my mind, as well as the reasons why I was doing it.

This really kept me going and it got rid of those roadblocks in my mind.

You might think, 'It's hard to visualise. It seems like a dream, not a reality that can happen.' Sure, but I advise you to picture it like you're watching a movie and you're the main actor. That would be exciting, right? And you're the hero in the movie.

Turning your struggle into a success story can be imagining that, for instance, you're being interviewed in a newspaper or on TV and the reporter asks you, 'Tell us how you were able to turn your struggles into an amazing, successful outcome in reaching your big goal.' (This could be fun to play around with ... try it!)

But don't just play around; do it for real and ask yourself how someone who's already been successful in doing something like your goal would have gotten past the mental roadblock. You be the reporter, so to speak.

'Your story is amazing Donna,' or, 'You have an amazing success story.' I come across this all the time when meeting people. I always refer to my *why*, like I did in the previous chapters, and then think of *how*: 'How do I get around this roadblock, this obstacle that may get in the way? How will I feel once I reach my goal?'

I know many people, me being one of them, who say it's hard to walk out the door, or get out of bed, or go to the gym, etc. some days, but the feeling afterwards is a great feeling and worth it in the end.

More than likely you will come across these moments when you have a mental roadblock and find it hard. The questions you need to ask yourself at this point are:

- Why am I doing this goal?
- How do I get around this roadblock?
- Who will be there when I reach my big goal?
- What will this moment look like through my eyes?

- Where will I be?
- How will I feel?
- How will this change me for the better?

But be prepared for roadblocks. You may not have control over some things.

Unfortunately, my next baby step goal for the 10 km challenge was delayed by injuries that I needed to rest from and get treatment for; of course this was frustrating, but something I needed to be patient with.

You may come across this yourself in your own goal journey, but please don't give up … it's okay to reset a date. Sometimes things happen in life that we really have no control over.

### #training #lesson
### February 2013 – Stress and uncertainty

In my journey from December to February, it was a stressful time at work. We knew there were changes being made and there were whispers about sending some of our work overseas where it would be cheaper for the business to move forward. We were all worried about our job, but were reassured in a team meeting that our jobs were safe. I was even given a special mention of the great work I had done in a short space of time, so I thought I was safe and stable in my role.

But in February there was mention among staff of other teams losing their jobs, one at a time exiting quietly, which made our team feel uncertain once again of the promise made to us earlier that year.

One morning it was made clear to us, I received a tap on my shoulder from my manager, asking me to meet in his office at 10.30am. I turned to Kate, my colleague sitting at her desk beside mine, looking worried at my knowing look that this was the dreaded meeting we were all hoping was a *rumour* for months. 'No Donna! You are great at your job, they wouldn't let go of you, don't worry.'

10.30 came, I entered the manager's office. He wasn't his cool friendly self, looking rather nervous. He explained the way the business was heading and how they had to let go of staff … blah blah blah … and yes as I thought, it was time for me to go. I actually felt for him. He couldn't look me in the eye and felt bad for me, telling me what a great job I did and that as I was the last employed there in his team, I was the first to go. It is funny looking back at this now, I was actually consoling him as I knew he could not look at me as he found this part of his role hard. He assured me that he was certain I would get another job without any problems and offered to be a referee for me, while leading me to his office door telling me it was time to leave now.

I went back to my desk, taking my belongings, with Kate looking at me in shock. I said goodbye to all the staff one at a time, receiving hugs and their well wishes and mostly looks of concern and disbelief, and some cheering me and saying they would continue to follow *Run Donna Run*.

I stood at the tram stop, wondering what my next move would be, and felt kind of numb. But at the same time I felt relieved. I had been stuck in a position of uncertainty for months, looking over my shoulder for that dreaded tap on my shoulder. It wasn't a great feeling. But I needed to keep moving forward.

This was a roadblock that could have easily led me to feel sorry for myself and get down on myself and distract me from my big marathon goal. But I didn't let it, realising that it was just a job, a job that I didn't even like! Looking at the bigger picture, it wasn't the end of my world. Now looking back, this was the push I needed, everything happens for a reason.

I actually gained more time to spend with my brother in Mildura, and a couple of months later I caught up with Kate who got me a position at her new job, so it was meant to be.

### #training #lesson
### March 2013 – My biggest roadblock

I heard a knock on my door late at night – this was unusual, and I was home alone.

'Who is it?' I called. I heard a faint voice, and it was my cousin Peter. I released the door chain and let him in, excited to see him as always but concerned at the look on his face. 'Hi Pete, are you okay?' I was surprised to see him at my door late at night.

He shook his head and stepped in the doorway, barely able to get his words out: 'It's Brian.'

I went to console him. 'Yes I know, it's hard, come in.'

'He's gone, Donna.'

'Where?' I responded.

He shrugged his shoulders, looking dismayed. 'He's gone. He died.'

'No!' I screamed. 'No! No!'

'I can't believe it either,' he said.

At that moment I felt the room spinning, holding on to Peter. He hugged me while I continually cried out, 'No, no,' in disbelief, sobbing like never before. 'I don't believe you.' I pulled back and stared at him, wanting an explanation. I only just saw Brian the day before.

'Yes Donna, I know … I don't believe it either. Your dad phoned me to come and tell you, and I just called him again when I parked the car here, to check if it was real.' This wasn't the response I wanted.

I'd only just gotten back from seeing him in Mildura the day before. My last words to him were, 'I'll see you soon,' as I was so sure I would. How could this happen?

Peter and I stood in each other's arms for an eternity, where I felt I was spinning fast, with uncontrollable tears and shock for most of that night, before I spoke to my Dad on the phone, questioning him for an explanation as to how this could happen.

This was a situation my dad could not explain in that moment; he couldn't fix it and make everything better. I could hear in his voice his helplessness to my questions … I passed the phone to Peter with no more words to find.

Eventually we rested, after repeating our words of disbelief; Peter fell asleep on the couch and I went to my bed. I left my lamp on and watched the ceiling spin, waiting to wake up… *this wasn't real, surely?* I thought. Still, nobody shook me to wake me up and tell me this was a bad dream.

I think after everything I have been through, my physical struggles, the stroke, diabetes, losing my job … that was nothing, compared to this. It was something that my willpower, my determination or even a pill could not fix. This was the most painful, difficult time for me and my family.

I took a break from training and spent time with my family in Mildura. Over that period of time, I was grateful to have support from extended family and friends … but I was still in disbelief. I may have switched off at times when people came to pay their respects. It felt strange, like it wasn't really happening. *Why are they visiting? Yes, it must have happened…*

I was asked a curious question by a couple of people in that period. 'Donna, will you still run the marathon in October?'

'Yes, of course! I'm not going to stop. Brian would want me to keep going,' I replied.

Brian was so encouraging of what I was doing, both with my personal challenge and fundraising. I remembered him saying to me, after he watched my 5.3 km run on video, how proud he was of me. I wanted to do this for him. I *needed* to do this for him. It was my reason *why* I needed to keep going with the marathon challenge.

I share this very personal story with you, to encourage you to keep going with your goal. It's okay to change the dates of your baby steps or even your big goal, but never lose focus on what you want to achieve in the end. Turn those mental blocks or misfortunes into a reason that carries you to keep pushing on and reach your goal.

I achieved my 10 km run challenge on 19 May in 91 minutes with an ankle injury, and a painful heart at Westerfolds ParkRun. Yes, I had times of struggle, even with the support from Chris along the way. I made this race about a few special people who had birthdays close to this event, my sisters Anne and Carla, and my mum and nephew. This always helped me push through. I was so grateful for Chris being there alongside me, his support and smile, and his commitment to me. I found out a lot more about him that day; it's funny the conversations that you have on a run.

> *'Never give up on something you really want. It's difficult to wait but it's more difficult to regret.'*
>     – Unknown

# Chapter 8

# Celebrating the Journey

Remembering to celebrate the steps we achieve along the way is just as important as the reward at the very end of your big goal.

Why? Because it keeps you going. It's important to enjoy the journey and see every hardship not as a negative, but as a positive once you've achieved it. I've come across people who are really tough on themselves and they're so stressed, they're not seeing the small achievements along the way. Sometimes that makes them negative and affects those around them too; it's not much fun to be around them, really.

The goal ends up being a chore rather than something exciting. If you keep it sounding like you're super-stressed and it ends up being a chore, not many people are actually going to support you; they'll see it as a negative rather than a positive, and may even try to talk you out of it.

Early in my training, I was turning into a stress-head at times. I was in Mildura on a hot summer Christmas break in 2012, on a training run with my brother in-law Ren – I had only been training for a month at this point. It was good to get out and train with him as we ran on a track along the Murray River, reminiscing about his younger years as a runner, and solving the problems of the world, as we often do … I grin as I write this. Ren said to me, 'Donna, remember to enjoy the journey, too.' The words that I needed to hear at the time.

I was fixated on the end result and my challenge. That's when I had to step back, break it down and create those baby steps – and actually be happy, once I'd achieved every baby step.

Some memories won't be as happy as others, perhaps. Most of mine were, because they were huge achievements to me. But you may find some people say, 'I wish I could have done that better.' Stop being hard on yourself and see it as a lesson; maybe this is a moment you could ask yourself, 'What can I do better in my next baby step? How can I have a better result than what I did before?'

Treat it like a game as well. Make it fun. It really builds confidence once you create your way to celebrate achieving each step, or even in just your training. It doesn't have to be the actual goal, but it can be little steps on the way through out your training and through your journey – like my 5.3 km run, for instance.

I tell people this a lot, when I can see that they're getting stressed and not enjoying the journey. As a result they may not get to the goal, because those are the times when you see people close to giving up.

I just really emphasise they need to take a 'chill pill'. Chill out; don't be so hard on yourself, because you're not seeing the achievements along the way. They may not be noticeable until you stop and think, or look back on your journaling notes, recordings or even pictures. Remember how I mentioned the importance of journaling earlier on in this book? There's a reason for my crazy ideas!

You can go to your mentor, coach, or your journal and review where you can improve. I did this, especially with my blood glucose testing for my diabetes. It taught me how to go about things the right way, so that I could train more successfully and not get that unnecessary 'worn out' feeling.

If you don't know much about diabetes, I'll explain: when your BG levels are high, you feel really tired and thirsty, and want to go to the toilet all the time. It just drains you of energy. When your BG level is low, similar effects can happen – not necessarily feeling thirsty, but just tired and shaky. Everybody's symptoms are different. Sometimes your head's not right – you can feel dizzy, even cranky and unfocused. There is a risk where you could go unconscious if you don't get sugar into the body on time. This is why I always carry jellybeans on me. They're my best friend.

That's just an example of what I found in my goal to be important to record. Everyone's goal is different, and you'll have your records, journals, charts, etc. to keep when reaching your goal. I highly recommend you do this.

Everyone looks forwards to a celebration or a reward, right? By rewarding yourself for each baby step, or even just the small goals along the way, this helps you to acknowledge the efforts you put into reaching your big goal and keeps you motivated to go for your next reward, and then the next …to get you to your finish line.

I really encourage this process, because I think a lot of times – not just in running, but with business or whatever your goal is – people just tend to get hard on themselves and not see the small achievements that are leading them to their big goal.

My marathon was eleven months away from when I started training. Some days it seemed like it was so far away, and other days it seemed like it was too close and I thought I needed to really catch up with my training, because I wasn't 100% confident that it was enough time for me. But my coaches reassured me, because they had the experience. Coaches and mentors can assure you and guide you to get the result. But for me it was still a long gap, so every small goal had a reward.

Take, for instance, the first goal of the 5.3 km run: I got a medal at the end and I felt so chuffed and proud of myself. I had a big smile for the rest of the day and I didn't take that medal off, not even when I went to a barbecue later that day. I was just so proud. I had been training for only a couple of months.

That's my point: even if it's the small steps, training for a small time, reward that small effort, because that's what gives you enthusiasm and excitement to keep going. I really believe that and it worked for me.

Another example: during my training I lived along a beachside in Elwood. At this particular place where I trained. Where I started and returned for my long runs, there was a gelato truck. I'd think, *I've got to complete this distance, because I want that gelato*. Just a simple thing like that was my reward. At the time I didn't particularly care about the diabetes, because I thought that after running such a long distance, a gelato's not going to do too much for my BG levels. That wasn't a big concern. But it was keeping the momentum and keeping me going. I'm just a big kid at the end of the day!

But for yourself, find something that you really enjoy. What do you like? How do you celebrate?

Find your 'special something' you like to do or receive. Some people say, 'I don't have time to celebrate.' Make it simple. I had time to eat a gelato. I also encourage people to celebrate by getting yourself something special that you don't often give yourself. Maybe it can be a physical product, a special dinner, or even a pizza night with your mates to brag about your achievement. That's awesome, having people around you, patting you on the back and keeping that excitement and momentum going – even in the early stages, that's what keeps you going and moving forward to your goal.

Get excited about your reward and tell someone. Don't make the excuse of saying, 'I don't have anyone to tell.' Write it down. Put it on your fridge, even: 'I'm working toward my reward of …'

It's a visual and an auditory thing, by putting it out there into the world. Acknowledge what you have done at the end of each week, or whenever, but make sure you do it often. Pat yourself on the back and don't be the person who's so hard on yourself, who ends up being a whiner who no one really wants to hang around with – that's not cool. (Just leave that for your coach's ears!)

My coach was good at cheering me on, if training alone. It's important to have someone cheering you on the sideline and steering you in the right direction when you lose your way. This in itself was a reward for me.

And then I've heard the excuses of, 'I don't have time, I can't think of each thing I've done to reward myself for, I'm too busy.' Busy schmizzy! Make this an important part of your routine in the steps that you make. Further in the book, where I've put the Baby Step Method, you will find a spot where you put your celebration or reward in the Baby Step Method table, whether it's big or small – it doesn't have to be expensive either.

The common excuses that I come across are, 'I don't have time; I don't have the money.' This is not the case in this situation. Make it something you look forward to and isn't a time waster or a big expense, because they're not big enough excuses for me and they shouldn't be for you either.

Even just choose a day, say every Sunday night, to write it down and see how productive you've been. Write down your new plan in the Baby Step Method table for that week or month and then you'll notice your progress for sure. As I've said with the journaling and so forth, you can look back at it and think, 'yeah, I have come a long way.'

I used to do video blogs; this was part of what I did for Run Donna Run for the people following me on my website or Facebook page. I'm glad I did that – even though I'm not a huge fan of doing videos, because I'm kind of clumsy in front of the camera. I'm not a natural, let's put it that way. But we did it to keep my gorgeous, keen followers in the loop with what was going on, because they were curious as to what was happening. Some were even inspired to train to run too. They were a great encouragement for me, and I'm still very grateful for that. But that's one way you could record your progress.

I remember doing voice recordings; some really tragic voice recordings too. There were a couple that I listen to now and think I wasn't really in a very good place that day, but I'm so proud of how I moved forward from that and I changed and shifted my mindset. You are allowed to have crappy days, that's natural, but just stepping out of that and thinking of something to reward yourself with will really keep you focused. I truly believe that.

Be good to yourself!

# Chapter 9

# Obstacle Challenge

I believe resilience – the ability to recover from setbacks, adapt well to change, and keep going when faced with adversity – is the key factor for *all* who achieve and get past obstacles in reaching their big goal.

For instance, when you get past the resilience factor, you know you can get through everything. It moves you forward and you gain confidence for the next challenge that you may face. You can see challenges as a threat or an opportunity for growth, so keeping a strong and resilient state of mind will get you through the obstacles that you'll face.

Also, be flexible with the obstacles that you may face. It doesn't necessarily have to be such a rigid, structured plan; sometimes we need to be flexible. This tests 'how bad you really want it'.

If you were to ignore the resilience factor, then you'd feel weak and overwhelmed from the obstacles that come up.

You'd feel low on self-esteem and give up easily on what you truly want. We don't want that. We want you to keep going and actually achieve your big goal.

The capacity to recover from a tough situation will test how resilient one is. This can be a learnt behaviour and doesn't necessarily mean one person is better than another; it's the choice that one makes. How one handles obstacles is the difference between the victor and the victim, the winner and the loser. I see it as a 'go for goals' attitude or 'sit on the couch' attitude. Most times, if we look at our strong *why*, there is no choice anyway.

How bad do you really want this?

### #training #lesson
### August, 2013 – The Devilbend *Fun Run* challenge

I was super-excited about my half-marathon challenge, though at the same time I did have concerns in the lead-up. My ankle had been giving me grief and was still sore at times when I ran on it, so I'd gotten Shaun to retape it. We had done all that we could, and I had put the training time in.

I've learnt along the way to accept what is ahead of me and do the best I can with what I have.

When I think about it, this is something I have done most of my life and even way back when I went through rehab, doing the best I can with what I have. You put the time and effort in and do the best you can, but sometimes the prep beforehand may slack off. This is where you notice the difference.

*Chapter 9 – Obstacle Challenge*

But the half-marathon challenge was too important for me to consider slacking off. I fought with my mind (and Shaun) at times when I needed to take time out to rest between training and recovery from uninvited injuries that truly annoyed me. The recovery period was testing my mental training.

But the half-marathon was a big challenge day – and one step closer to the full marathon. I made a choice not to focus on the dodgy ankle, but just to do what I could in prep to maintain my staying power. There was no way anything would get between me and the finish line.

I was calm that morning, even after a restless night, having breakfast advised by Chris along with Enisa and Rebecca (my diabetes team) helping me prepare for the running distance of 21.1 km for a person with type 1 diabetes. I collected the bag of goodies I prepared the night before, including: my blood test monitor, a banana for after the run, a water bottle, jellybeans, and other endurance snacks I had tested in my long training runs. I looked at the bag thinking I over-prepared, but it's better than having under-prepared, and I had my friends to look after my goodies for me.

But this half-marathon was a far longer distance than my usual runs, so just to be cautious as a person with type 1 diabetes, I planned to carry a belt with a few goodies just in case. This time I also wore a CGM (continuous glucose monitor). This was a real test in preparation for the marathon challenge, to know when I may experience peaks and troughs and how to level them out where my BG and energy levels were concerned. This can be a juggling act, but one we were trying to refine to get me to the home run with no balls dropped, so to speak. I'm sure any person with diabetes can relate to this.

After a long drive, my friends and I arrived at the event; the excitement was all around. This is what I love about running events: everyone is buzzing and excited for each other, sharing which race they are entering, their training stories and personal best times they aim to beat.

I took in the excitement and looked for a spot to test my BG level before the run. I was happy with the result; *A good level before a long run*, I thought – a little high, but only by a tiny amount that I was sure I would run off in time anyway.

Chris found us with a huge smile once again and I was grateful to have my support team there for me on this fresh early morning, all smiling and excited with me. Chris promised to meet me at some stage during the run, planning to film me but also to offer support and check up on me as a nutrition advisor. I had been showing a few concerns getting through the longer runs recently, so he said he'd meet me at some point with my BG monitor too.

Quickly munching on an energy ball, I was among the enthusiastic pack of crazy runners – yes, me being one of them! Waving to my awesome support team, I was off and running.

This was exciting, I was actually participating in a half-marathon! Slowly moving forward, I heard a voice running beside me: 'You're Donna, right?'

*Chapter 9 – Obstacle Challenge*

I turned to see a huge smile on a friendly face. 'Yes, how did you know?' I replied in surprise, not recognising her.

'You're Run Donna Run! I follow your Facebook page and I read your story on the race event website, great story!'

'Thanks! Is this your first half-marathon?' I asked her.

'Yeah,' she replied with excitement.

My ankle was already giving me a slight pain; maybe I should have taken more painkillers, but it was too late. I had to keep going and suck it up. Revealing to my new friend that I had an ankle issue, she claimed she was getting over an injury too. This made me realise there were so many among this crowd of runners who all carried their own stories. But everyone was supportive of one another and holding each other high.

I found a feeling of positive overwhelm on this particular run. I realised that many of these fellow runners knew who I was and had read my interview article that the event organisers had put on their website. I was overwhelmed by the encouragement I received by people passing me by and yelling out my name: 'Run Donna run!' 'Go Donna!' 'Well done Donna!' 'Great effort!' I hadn't even finished yet! There were runners high-fiving as they went past. I truly felt blessed to have so much encouragement; it blew me away and kept me smiling all the way.

Writing this now brings tears to my eyes; I know

it may sound silly, but it is a wonderful memory of true camaraderie, encouragement and enthusiasm that I will remember forever with a big smile on my face and a glow in my heart.

It turned into a beautiful day with the sun out. I had a drink at every stop and took energy drinks they were offering at aid stations. I was in two minds as to know how much energy drinks to consume (considering their sugar content); they weren't large cups so I thought they may help and that I'd run it off anyway.

This half-marathon track was a circuit that we needed to cover twice, and a little extra, to complete the 21.1 km distance. I could feel three super-fast runners come from behind me; these guys couldn't be slower than me! They were obviously on their second round and they were the three leading the race. These guys were awesome and on a mission! The third guy with blonde spikey hair past me and turned over his shoulder, yelling, 'I read your story last night, great story Donna … keep going!' This guy was running a race but took the time to encourage me along his way, which I found to be awesome.

I knew I was heading close to the 10 km mark as I could hear music and the sound of people cheering. I came around a corner to an open space with the buzzing of the starting area. I could see Chris and my friends cheering me with big smiles. I stopped to check my BG reading and gave a quick response to Chris's questions: 'I'm feeling a lot of pain in my ankle when landing on my foot Chris…'

*Chapter 9 – Obstacle Challenge*

My BG read 16. 'Oh, this is why I'm feeling so exhausted already! Maybe I had too much energy drink?' When my BG is high, I feel tired and out of energy, but I was determined to move on and complete this challenge.

I stood there with my support team, questioning myself and wondering what Dr Matt or Rebecca (my dietician) would say, deciding whether to keep going or give myself a correction dose of insulin to bring me to a good BG level. But I thought back to when I had trained hard sessions with Shaun and wondered why my BG levels would go high. Enisa (my diabetes educator) said it was from my adrenaline and not to give a correction dose of insulin, as it usually comes down again naturally … but I was only halfway through, would it come down soon?

I decided not to take any insulin and just kept going, with a promise from Chris that he would meet me during the second half to do another BG reading. So I made the decision and thought, *I must keep going.*

Heading off to the start line again under the big banner and past the cheering crowd, I heard Kriss on my right 'Run Donna Run'; my wonderful friend came all this way to cheer me on. I was shocked to see her there, yelling out to her, 'I'm only halfway! You're here too soon, they're all that way!' while pointing toward my team and Chris.

Round two, here I come! I headed around the wide open space, then past Chris and my friends again before entering a path that had a ditch to run over to get on the new track. I carefully managed to avoid a 'Donna trip' when another runner ran towards me, obviously on his second circuit, cheering me on then landing splat on the ground – he fell hard! I stopped to see if he was alright, and if he wanted me to get first aid, but he got up quick, assuring me he was fine and racing in the direction of our joint goal, the finish line. He was on a mission and there was no stopping him! We all were …

Straight after that, my shoe lace busted – damn! I seemed to go through so many shoelaces lately! So I stopped and sat at the side on the ditch edge of the track to fix up my shoe, especially to hold my leg brace in place inside my shoe. This wasn't the time to run with a loose shoe or no leg brace. I managed to fix the situation and kept on going.

I now saw many people coming in the opposite direction; I knew I wasn't the fastest runner on this track, but that was not the point for me. Everyone had their own story and own goal. For me it was all about completing it and if I didn't get there in the speed of light, that was fine too. Even though I like to make goal times for myself, I did this to keep focused – not only on the day, but all through my training. Sometimes my goals may be considered too big by some, but this is what keeps me going and hey, a marathon is freakin' *huge* but I was still going for it!

I met another awesome young woman, probably about twenty years of age, running toward me, yelling excitedly, 'Donna, I was so inspired by your story. I'm running today because of you!'

Chapter 9 – Obstacle Challenge

'Awesome, well done!' was my response. But in my mind, my response was, Wow! Are you serious? *I inspired you to come and run a half-marathon today? Really?*

That was a golden moment for me; to think little seven-year-old Donna could make a difference and inspire others ... wow!

There were very few people around me now; this was the part that would test my mentality. No cheering, no Chris, nothing but cows along the way. This was truly a beautiful place to be. If I weren't running a half-marathon I would've wanted to stop, take photos and pause to enjoy the peaceful view. But there was no time for that.

Heading toward another aid station, there were two cheery volunteers (gotta love them) encouraging me and offering drinks. I took water this time; I didn't want to risk the chance of raising my BG levels further. And there, popping out of nowhere, was Chris my saviour, with my BG monitor – awesome! Pricking my finger, I did a test and it was back on track at a good level – I was happy with that. I waved with gratitude and kept moving forward, leaving them behind. I heard Chris invite the volunteers to the fundraiser dinner I was organising. I grinned to myself thinking, *he's a gem.*

I went on further, now hobbling more than usual from the pain in my ankle and hip. I was losing the sound of humans to what seemed like the never-ending yellow brick road. Where was the Wizard? Toto? The Tin Man? And whoever else is in that support gang ... is it the Mad Hatter?

Was I getting my stories mixed up? *OMG! Snap out of it Donna!*

I had to think: what kept me focused when training, when things got tough? Yes, that's right! My mantra from Julie: 'There's no such thing as can't!'

Looking up ahead, I saw a tiny man standing by the pole where we had to turn around – okay, awesome! That's where I get to turn and eventually head over the finish line!

*Keep focused, think of the finish line Donna*, the voice in my head kept telling me.

*Yeah, but can we get there sooner?* asked the other voice …

*Here comes a runner, coming toward me! A human! I'm not the only one on this track!* Moving closer, I realised it was the friendly smiling woman who spoke to me right at the beginning of the race, the woman who knew me from my page! I was so pleased to see her. She was struggling too, but she was still in the game.

'Is that the pole where we turn around to come back?' I asked her with enthusiasm.

'No, you have to go up further and do a bit extra on this round.'

Oh bummer! 'How are you going?' I asked her, realising I don't know her name.

'Sore, but okay … I have to finish this. How are you?'

*Chapter 9 – Obstacle Challenge*

'Really sore, I'm now struggling here,' I said, pointing to my groin. She stopped to show me stretches that would help. Grateful for her help, I thanked her and encouraged her to keep going – I didn't want to hold her back from her goal.

'I'll see you at the finish line, Donna,' she said, running off with a smile.

'What's your name?'

'Lou.'

'Run Lou, run!' I yelled, cheering her on, and kept going. I was more determined to get to the pole and do that extra bit, so I could turn back and see her at the finish line … and my friends and Chris.

Making it to the pole, the volunteer pointed me in the direction of an off-road track that was rough and sludgy at times. I really had to take it easy on this track and walk it; there was no way I could possibly do more damage to my ankle any further. Now I was on my own again, with the conflicting voices going on in my head.

I was chanting out loud, 'The power is in me, the power is in me, the power is in me …' in puffed out breaths. 'Keep going Donna!'

I now reminded myself of my *why*. There were so many reasons to complete this challenge!

I was raising funds for the RCH. I was out here in hope of inspiring and encouraging others. I had people following my journey and encouraging me every day, and Shaun and Chris.

I was doing this for my encouraging friends and family. There was my brother Brian whom I kept in my mind. This particular race was also for my sister Toni, who just had her birthday a few days ago.

This race was for me too; it was a huge personal challenge for me. I had plenty of reasons to keep going.

I wondered what the time was. It didn't matter. All I needed to do was keep moving forward in any way possible … run … hobble … repeat …

I stopped for more water with the cheery volunteers again. They were yelling, 'Run Donna, run!' this time – obviously Chris told them about the Run Donna Run challenge. I was happy to see them, that was for sure. I ran off admiring the wonderful views again and enjoying seeing the cows again too… and then Chris popped out of nowhere.

'Crap, you scared me!' I said smiling.

'How are you going, Donna?'

'I'm really sore here,' I said, pointing to my groin. 'I feel like I've had rough sex for a week!' We chuckled and kept going.

'You're on the last stretch now, Donna.'

Not at a great speed now, to the point of great struggle. We saw volunteers packing up the last aid station. Brett, a friend and one of the event organisers, ran up to us and back alongside us to support me. 'You're doing great, Donna.'

*Chapter 9 – Obstacle Challenge*

'Thanks Brett, just feeling really sore now. I would have liked to have gone faster. This has been a great day though, well done! Everyone has been so supportive, I am blown away by their enthusiasm and encouragement.' I then asked the guys, 'What's the time?'

Chris checked his watch. Bummer, it was past the time I predicted and even more than what Shaun predicted.

This was no time for being annoyed with my time; I was here and about to complete a half-marathon. That was good enough for me.

Now I'd reached the bridge that led back to the finish line. 'You've got some fans waiting for you, Donna,' Brett said.

I could see a young boy and two blonde women cheering.

'Oh, they waited, this is Thomas!' I explained to Chris and Brett. 'And his mum Annitta and her friend Laura, they waited all this time!'

'You have to pick up your pace now, Donna.' Chris jeered me on.

I laughed. 'I know! I am really struggling though, guys …'

We picked up our pace. I was so pleased to see them in the flesh. We'd only had contact through my Facebook page; this was such a buzz for me. To have Thomas, who was only nine years old and a past RCH patient, run with me … we all said our quick hellos and kept running.

There were still a few people left, but those who were there cheered me on. I was so grateful for their cheers of encouragement.

Chris, Brett, Annitta and Laura slowed down to give me my moment to cross the finish line. 'Okay Thomas, are you running over with me?' Of course he was keen and ran ahead as I halted just a few steps before the finish line. My legs felt like jelly. I could hear my friends now cheering me on too, along with the event organiser: 'Keep going Donna!' What could have been a second felt like a minute-long pause as I revived my jelly legs. Avoiding collapsing on the ground, I made it over the line! I did it! I don't know why I paused right before the finish line, but I got over the finish line and achieved my goal.

Hugs and cheers were all around. I didn't even look at the timer, it was kind of a blur … But there was Lou with her medal around her neck and a big smile and hug. She made it and waited at the finish line for me too! I was so proud she made it and grateful she kept her promise to see me at the finish line.

Photos were taken, fruit was handed to me with drinks and even a first aid volunteer offered painkillers, which I gladly took.

This was a huge day for me; I couldn't lose the smile on my face, even though I was in so much pain. 'Do I really have to walk to the car now?' I debated out loud. We all chuckled but I managed to hobble, way more than usual, with a half-marathon medal I wore around my neck for the rest of the day. I walked to the car without falling, still smiling.

The power is in me, hey?

I've heard people say, 'I want my goal so much, but sometimes it just gets too hard.' This half-marathon challenge was hard, but knowing how much I wanted it, my reasons why and reminding myself of my mantras all helped me get to the finish line. I recommend you make a mission statement, like your business or workplace or even at school. There's a mission statement at these places that we're obliged to stand by and work under, right? If you're finding it really tough, why don't you create your own mission statement? It will move you forward and keep you confident for the next challenge you may face.

> 'It's not whether you get knocked down, it's whether you get up.'
> – Vince Lombardi

### #training #lesson
### December 2012 – Injury obstacles

I tried to hide my training injuries from my parents when I stayed with them over the Christmas break in 2012, even though I shared this publicly with people around the world on Facebook. Thank goodness my parents aren't on Facebook. My mum had always been encouraging but I didn't want them to react with concern, or give Dad more reason to doubt this challenge.

There were times when I'd go to stay at their home; with a staircase to and from the bedroom, it had been a struggle to climb or come down the stairs depending on the injury. I tried doing this secretly, without them seeing. I felt like a seven year old sneaking to the pantry to get a cookie from the tin, but instead I was sneaking to the freezer to grab my ice pack to soothe my knee, ankle, hip – whatever injury I had at the time – while grabbing a glass of water to sneak a painkiller or two.

I know this sounds silly at forty-two years of age, but this has been my life concern: to lessen the worry from my parents of 'Donna the sick child'. Now I was facing this marathon challenge. It contradicted my concern for not wanting to worry my parents … I don't think I was doing a very good job.

It was hard work to get to where I am today. This applies to my parents too. They were the team leaders for my fight for success – for living, walking, talking, and maintaining good health. For the time, patience, support, concern and encouragement they contributed to my transformation.

My personal contribution was determination, self-motivation, impatience and frustration (at times) towards the physical challenges that I needed to face to get me here, and overcoming the mental challenges (I'm guilty of always being a person who likes something done yesterday).

So I didn't need to face a marathon challenge. This was a choice, some would say a crazy challenge that I had placed on myself.

I am a big believer of there always being room for improvement, and that applies to me physically and mentally. With all that in mind, there was one major concern I put to Shaun at the beginning. 'I don't want to go backwards, Shaun. Could this distance cause me to have major injuries? Put it this way ... I don't want to end up back in a wheelchair.' I knew that the wheelchair comment was a little farfetched, but I wanted to get my point across to Shaun.

Shaun assured me it wouldn't cause major injuries. 'Sure, you will feel sore, ask anyone who runs a marathon. You will go through pain, but it won't last forever.'

Questioning my flow of injuries during training, he stated that I was using different muscles from movements that I hadn't experienced for many years. I was waking up muscles that had been asleep for thirty-four years.

Shaun is always convincing; sometimes I think he should be a politician. He has not only turned out to be a great coach to me, but more. I know as a regular coach he wouldn't normally have the constant contact that I have pushed on him, so I am very grateful for his coaching and friendship to this day.

I sometimes wondered if he secretly had the 'Oh no, Donna!' moments, when he heard of another injury notch I had added to my belt. But he always seemed so cool and encouraging and direct with instructions. This is exactly what I needed. Shaun always had some obscure saying or quote that he came out with that was not always understood by me, but I was grateful for the effort all the same.

*'Pain is inevitable. Suffering is optional. Say you're running and you think, "Man this hurts, I can't take it anymore." The hurt part is an unavoidable reality, but whether or not you can stand anymore is up to the runner himself.'*

– Haruki Murakami

## Chapter 10

# Winning Language

I often advise people to talk to themselves as if they were talking to their best friend. This may sound strange at first, but it helps get your mental and physical state off to a good start.

What benefits does this positive language give you? You feel good. It really helps when you're struggling and it motivates you to keep going. It makes you grateful. It reminds you to be kind to yourself and encouraging; sometimes we can be really hard on ourselves. Giving yourself those rewards, celebrating and being kind in the way you talk to yourself – that's what I mean by the winning language. Talk to yourself like you would to your best friend.

What would you feel if you didn't do that? You'd feel down on yourself. You'd lose self-belief and confidence, creating negative energy. If you keep being so negative and down, people don't want to be around you and that creates negative energy towards your big goal, and you'll never get encouragement to reach your big goal. People will want you to stop going for it because they'll see it as something that maybe isn't a good thing for you. But you know it's a great thing for you, because it's a big dream that you've always wanted to achieve.

So our self-talk is very important, because it's with us every day.

'You're sounding a bit crazy, Donna.' Maybe, but we talk to ourselves all the time.

Those thoughts in your mind are like a number of voices in your head sometimes. When we think encouraging and motivating thoughts toward ourselves, then we see results in our ability to reach our big goal.

Be your best friend. You may say, 'I don't understand how to be my best friend, but that doesn't make sense.' Think of the conversation you may have had with a good friend where they were struggling with something. What words of advice or encouragement did you give them? These words you need to give to yourself.

I use the example of when I started training in November 2012. I was being hard on myself, because I am the kind of person who, like I said, likes to have things done yesterday and I can get impatient with myself at times. My coach can confirm that too.

Anyway, there were days when I worked really hard, but still there were days when I would struggle, so it wasn't always smooth sailing (especially at the beginning). So I'd really get down on myself for slowing down to walk instead of running.

But that was just the beginning. I would have these horrible thoughts in my mind, talking to myself. *Come on Donna, you're being slack … blah blah blah* – criticising myself.

When I thought about this and I had a conversation with my coach, he said to me, 'You need to talk to yourself in an encouraging way.' I totally agree. That's what really helps you get to your goal, through the baby steps.

I understand not everyone is going to have a mentor or a coach – whether that's a life coach, business or adventure coach – for every goal they want to achieve. So the important thing to remind ourselves of here is that it all starts with you. How are you talking to yourself?

If I was to go do a training session, running along with a friend of mine, and she said, 'Look, Donna, I have to slow down right now, can I just walk?' I'm not going to blast her and tell her she's being slack. Would you do that to your best friend? I don't think so. I would say, 'Okay, that's fine, are you in any pain?' If she's not then, 'That's fine, we can walk – you're moving forward and that's a good thing.' It's as simple as that. It's not giving a big lecture to her. You would be encouraging, telling her how good she's doing and the distance she has done already, maybe even distracting her with conversation on what a great day it has been, etc.

Whether it's walking or running, there have been people I've coached or lead in my adventure challenges who start out struggling and say to me, 'I've only done a little bit of running Donna, I'm only walking, running, walking, running,' I tell them, 'That's great because you're moving forward!' Often we can be guilty of being hard on ourselves. My simple advice: 'Stop it!'

When using winning language, I find quotes have really helped me. One in particular was Julie's mantra: 'There is no such thing as can't.' That's stayed in my mind ever since that day and I've used it a lot when times are tough, and I've been through bad times – not just physically but emotionally too.

Even if you're not the type of person to put things on the wall or your fridge, if you have it in your mind it will help you with your winning language. I know people who just repeat their mantras out loud or in their head. I was doing that sometimes when I was running: 'There's no such thing as can't, no such thing as can't.' I kept my motivation up by using those quotes in a positive way.

A number of years ago, before the marathon challenge, I also created another quote that is a favourite of mine: 'The power is in me.' This has a lot to do with choice. I remember thinking this and not even saying it out loud. It was a choice that I had once, when I could sit on the edge or actually dive in and give it a go. *The power is in me, I have so much power, I live in a country where we have many choices that we can make, and we're free to make decisions.* I used it a lot too when I was training.

Especially in reacting to obstacles, there are choices we make. With obstacles and resilience, we can easily curl up on the couch and just stay there, being the victim. But that's not going to get us to our goals. That's why I believe these quotes can help us in those tough moments.

You might be thinking now, 'I can't think of a quote that I like.' The internet is awesome; I advise you to look up 'inspiring quotes' on any topic or goal you have. You'll be surprised what you find – there's lots of stuff online. But make sure it's 'inspiring quotes' and use the words 'inspiring', 'motivating', etc. – words that are going to keep you going, when you do your search. There are plenty of quotes out there that are negative as well, we don't want those.

An important practise that is commonly forgotten, when going for goals or just in life in general, is the habit to show gratitude. I had so much support and I'm still very grateful to people who gave me support in various areas throughout my marathon goal journey.

## Chapter 10 – Winning Language

I'm forever grateful to my coaches for my physical training and their support. But I also had great support just in encouragement from people who followed me, such as through social media, and letters from supporters. I had people create events for my fundraising goal, and people attended events that I created – I am super-grateful for that. People sponsored me as well. So always show gratitude; I truly believe this should not be forgotten. For example, I show people gratitude by simply thanking them and letting them know how I truly appreciate them and their support, and how important their involvement has been within my project. I also share this with others to let people know of their amazing support or the work they've put in, and help promote their skills.

At the end of a speaking event, I enjoy it when people come up and share their stories with me. It's just gorgeous; I love that at the end of my talks. I usually invite people to come up and talk to me and even share what their goal is, or if they're struggling with something.

At one particular event, two people came up to me, a mother and daughter, to say hi. I remember the mother saying to me, 'My daughter and I were just talking about how people like yourself ... who have been through some sort of struggle ... we notice that they come out to be inspiring people. Why is that? What do you put that down to? Can you tell us why and how you're like that?'

I said to them, 'Maybe it's because we're determined.' Then I said straight after that, 'It's gratitude! I think the main thing is gratitude. Because we're grateful for where we've come from to where we are now.' I'm speaking for myself here, but I see it a lot in people who've been through adversity.

When I think now of gratitude, it makes me think of a story about a boy named Brendan.

## #training #lesson
## 1979 – Brendan's story

I still don't fully know what diagnosis Brendan had, but he was clearly in a serious condition back in 1978/79. He was secluded from us children in Ward 6. Our room in Ward 6 had children coming and going – some stayed longer than others. Some we got to know more than others.

Ward 6 was for children with blood conditions. It was bright, with walls painted white and pictures stuck on the walls for the kids. It was like any other hospital but filled with children, all with their own stories but with blood conditions. It was not always bright.

Our room could fit six beds in it, three beds on either side facing each other as you entered the room. The two walls either side of the doorway had windows halfway up to the ceiling; this meant staff could see what was going on in our room easily, but it also meant we could see them too.

Huge windows on the wall opposite the doorway brought in plenty of light. During the day we had a view of the green oval where the helicopter landed to bring in more sick children like us. It was peaceful to see the stars at night, reminding us there was a whole universe outside of Ward 6.

Even though we were surrounded by glass, we still had our privacy when needed, by a white curtain hanging from a rail above our beds. This was our private cocoon.

The rooms for the patients were all on one side of the passageway, and on the other side were

Chapter 10 – Winning Language

other rooms closed off for staff use, bathrooms, a kitchenette and a room where they did private examinations on patients (that room I didn't like – it always meant they'd jab my veins, which weren't easy to find). And there was one special glass room directly opposite us with Brendan in it.

We considered Brendan a part of our 'team', even though there was a passageway dividing us. He had his own white curtain that slid across his window when he needed his private time.

We all waved to tiny Brendan as he got more pale and frail each day. Brendan had been in Ward 6 for a while now, but I don't recall exactly how long … minutes turned into hours, hours turned into days, and days turned into weeks in Ward 6. He was a similar age to me, but I wasn't really sure – as many of us were quite frail, it was hard to guess. He still showed a smile and a spark in his eyes responding to all who acknowledged him. We would sometimes go close to his window to wave and smile, when I could get out from my bed.

The nursing staff was always very good with us. Some were loud, some were jolly and smiled more than others, but they all showed they cared in their own way and were great with all of us, including our families.

The cleaners in Ward 6 had become familiar faces and shared their smiles too, not wanting to get in our way. Some did not even share the same language, but all shared a nod with a smile, and knew how to say hello. They were a part of our day to day lives. One cleaning man brought a wheely table from another ward to extend to its highest level, so Brendan could see his cards and flowers through his glass cocoon.

Brendan would smile and giggle at the attempts made by all who frequently passed his decorative window – filled with pictures, drawings and decorations stuck high on the outside of his window – to remind him of the care and thoughts that so many people had for him. The cleaners would smile, walk backwards or make silly faces.

One funny cleaner walked past each day taking each step lower, appearing to disappear with only a hand remaining in sight, waving to Brendan through his window. This always made us all burst into laughter. But we could not hear his laugh, we only saw it on his tiny face with eyes so blue, they seemed to glimmer to light up his pale face.

Brendan's only window looked out to the passageway, and to us in our room of six beds. We all made sure, when we could, that he was not forgotten, as he was a big part of our group. This was the strong bond that most of us formed, especially those of us who were there for a longer time.

One morning my mum entered Ward 6, and Brendan wasn't in his room. She turned to me and the five other children in the room to see my look of worry.

'Where's Brendan?' she asked.

*Chapter 10 – Winning Language*

I shook my head. 'The alarm went off last night with the light flashing above his door!' I spoke in a fast confused voice. 'Mum, I don't know where he is – I don't know, Mum!'

'He is probably having tests done. Remember when you had to be taken to have a CT scan at the other hospital?' Mum answered, sounding doubtful of her own explanation. She tried to change the mood in the room with an activity to entertain (and distract) me for the rest of the morning. She was good at that.

Later that afternoon, a ghost-like figure walked into Ward 6; her face was as pale as the crisp white gown she usually wore. Only this time, Brendan's mother wasn't wearing her usual gown. She had no hair cover, revealing her mousy brown hair bun that looked messed. Brendan's mother had a faded expression and dark circles under her eyes that looked like dried up puddles, where tears once lay. Immaculately dressed as always, but hardly noticeable most times due to the white coat, mask and hair cover that she wore.

It didn't matter; Ward 6 was a place where it didn't matter what style of clothing you wore or your background, race or religion. We were all the same and had the same intention: to get well and go back home. We hoped it for ourselves and for every other kid in Ward 6.

Brendan's mum walked toward his table outside of his room, full of thoughts and sentiments, and slowly opened each card to read with a faraway expression. She delicately placed each card in her brown carry bag, one at a time, after reading each message. She hadn't looked up or even realised that people existed around her.

My eyes were fixed on Mum, wanting to know where Brendan was. But instead she placed her finger on my lip. Seeing Brendan's mum and what she was doing, I guessed what had happened from the alarm light flashing the night before.

I quickly put my head down and kept colouring in my book with my determined left hand, while taking sneaking glances at Brendan's mum and then at my mum. It was a difficult task to wait and stay silent with so many questions unanswered, and an overly curious mind.

Brendan's mother completed collecting her son's cards and slowly picked up one of the flower bouquets that was about to die, placing it delicately into the rubbish bin under the sink nearby. She resembled a ballerina practicing her warm-up stretches in slow motion, removing the coloured paper decorations from the outside of Brendan's glass room that we made in occupational therapy for him. She removed the photos, the posters, the decorative thoughts that kept Brendan in touch with the outside world of his glass cocoon.

Brendan's mother walked ever so carefully, carrying each of Brendan's many flower arrangements, taking them to the other bed tables in our room for other children. There was one bunch with yellow carnations that only looked like they had a day left to live. Another small cheerful-looking bunch she placed on Tom's bedside table opposite me. She then slowly carried another bright bouquet over to the unattended nurse's desk, removing the small card attached to it. I wondered if they would notice or even know who left them there.

It amazed me thinking of the time that Brendan was in Ward 6; it seemed like a long time to me, and he was still receiving flowers and cards from loved ones. Brendan was special and it saddened me to think we never got to hear his voice.

There were no words spoken or sounds made while she moved around the room with little effort. This had always been her way in the time we had known Brendan's mother; she had always been so gracious. Even during the long hours of caring for her son, nothing had ever seemed to be an effort, even when doing things for others.

All parents did the same for each child in our room, especially if their family wasn't around. Even though Brendan was across the hall in his own special room, and we weren't able to help him directly, we all still smiled and waved and shared our look of concern when needed; we'd let the staff know if we thought he looked uncomfortable or needed attention, if his mum wasn't there (although she was there most hours).

I don't know if anyone else could see what Brendan's mum was doing with his flowers. She appeared to be unnoticed by others. Is this what happens when you've been there, like part of the furniture, for so long in Ward 6?

Brendan's mum picked up the last flower arrangement, the freshest and largest of the lot. I turned my head briefly to look at my book. Then I looked up in surprise to find her standing right in front of me, placing the beautiful fresh flowers carefully on my bed table, next to where I was doodling. Mum quickly stood up to respond when Brendan's mum interrupted her desperate moment of speechlessness.

'These are for Donna, the freshest flowers that will live longer than the rest. Brendan would have wanted Donna to have them.' Her fixed look met my Mum's welled eyes, as firm as the grasp that she held on her wrist. With no further words, she half-smiled at my sad wondering eyes, and quickly turned with her hand holding her bowed forehead. Swiftly collecting her belongings, she followed the green floor line and exited the door of Ward 6 for the very last time, leaving us with a bittersweet bouquet. A scent of a sweet life taken away from the grasp of a mother's last hope.

At that moment when she left the room, the room was no longer bright. A cloud passed over the sun, and dimmed the light in our room immediately, as she left us looking at Brendan's empty room, with no greeting cards, flowers or decorations hanging on his window. Just an empty wheely table sitting outside of his room that looked out of place. It was not always bright in Ward 6.

With the loss of Brendan, this moment taught me the meaning of gratitude: to be grateful for the support from the people around me and for my life that I was close to losing – even if I struggled with tasks now that came easy to me before the stroke. I wish the lesson were not so grave. It still leaves a lump in my throat telling you this story.

## Chapter 10 – Winning Language

*'When it comes to life, the critical thing is whether you take things for granted or take them with gratitude.'*
  – Gilbert K. Chesterton

I have an exercise you can do with gratitude. I definitely recommend this one. Before going to sleep at night, think of seven things you are grateful for from that day. Say it out loud or in your mind. Just acknowledge it. I always do it when I've got my head on the pillow, before I go to sleep. *I'm grateful for the legs I have to carry me. I'm grateful for my bed, my family, to have a roof over my head; I'm grateful for my friends, or whatever has happened in my day.* And so on.

Think about what you are grateful for, whether it's big or small. Make sure you acknowledge what you have; this is a really big thing to move you forward, especially when you're struggling.

So with what I said earlier about the running: once I thought about it, I was kind to myself and thinking, *Hey, okay, I'm walking right now, but I was running before, and then I'm going to run and then I'm going to walk ... and that's fine. Just keep it up, keep moving forward. Once upon a time I wasn't able to walk, I wasn't able to run.* Putting that in my mind makes me grateful and keeps me moving forward.

I encourage you to use my running example too, of training beside a friend who's struggling. What do you say to them? Use this in your challenge. It may not be running, it may be something else, but do this as a daily exercise.

Whenever something comes up in your head and you're being really negative to yourself and hard on yourself, be your best friend.

*'Man often becomes what he believes himself to be. If I keep on saying to myself that I cannot do a certain thing, it is possible that I may end by really becoming incapable of doing it. On the contrary, if I have the belief that I can do it, I shall surely acquire the capacity to do it even if I may not have it at the beginning.'*
– Mahatma Gandhi

## Chapter 11

# Your Roadmap to the Finish Line

This is the action part – goody!

This is an easy, step by step process where you won't feel overwhelmed. When you go through all the insights, processes and personal experiences I've delivered in these chapters, you will also see it as an adventure or game when using my Baby Step Method, and most of all you'll feel proud when achieving each step. It simplifies things. It creates steps to keep it doable and keep you motivated.

You won't want to give up when using this method. You'll feel great when you've achieved your results. You won't stay feeling stuck or depressed, believing you will never achieve your big goal. That negative attitude doesn't serve you or your family and friends, and I don't want that for you.

If you find things are difficult, it will be easier to give up and make excuses, and actually believe your excuses. You'll end up having fear and an 'it looks too hard' attitude. We need to get past this and achieve, don't we?

Using baby steps with your big goals is the most doable approach I've found, and I've used it to help others gain results and achieve their big goals.

I used it myself in my big goal, going from running thirty steps to completing a full marathon. The knowledge you have now from reading the previous chapters, and knowing what I've achieved and even helped others achieve, will give you a 'no limits' mentality to reach further and succeed in goals you may have steered away from, because in the past you thought it was too difficult.

How do we go about the Baby Step Method? You write a plan, create your steps and determine the end result needed for each step. This includes putting dates and times on goals. For example, a big goal for losing weight might be, 'I want to weigh 60 kg by 20 January 2018.'

The first baby step could be, 'I want to lose one kilogram a week, for four weeks.' This will increase after four weeks; maybe the goal will be more intense, to lose more weight in a shorter period. This is where I would seek help from experts, to be specific about your goal.

Is the above goal doable? It's saying specifically what the amount is that you want to lose. It's not just saying, 'I want to lose weight.' It's being specific and it's putting a time on it. Excellent.

People might say, 'I'm not good at drawing up plans and rosters and routines.' Well, that's what the Baby Step Method is about, and you'll see it at the end of this book. It's all set up for you. But you need to put your own individual plans in place, because everybody's goal is different.

You could get help – for example, from someone who's lost weight already, a friend, or a PT who can say what's achievable. Be realistic: go to a gym three days a week, go to a nutritionist, that sort of thing. Put times on this too – what period of time are you spending at the gym at each session? Make a plan by using the Baby Step Method, and make it achievable.

If you're a person who doesn't like a written plan, you can even draw pictures or use photos, or make recordings of reminders telling you what to do for that day or week. But don't get lazy with this – that's why I really recommend the Baby Step Method table, as it's set out for a period of time that you need to follow to complete each step, and if you stick it somewhere you can see every day (e.g. your fridge, above your desk, etc.), that's even better! It's a constant reminder!

Be specific with your time and goal – that's the most important thing. But also be specific with the small goals that get you to your *big* end achievement.

Example: The baby steps of my marathon goal.

- Step 1: 5.3 km fun run.
- Step 2: The 10 km race.
- Step 3: The half-marathon.
- Step 4: The full marathon – the *big* scary goal.

I took these steps and gradually increased the distance and intensity. When you're seeking advice from someone, make sure it's doable, but also increase your intensity. The greater the challenge, the more you work for it, and that's exciting!

I really believe that. Because once you've had a few weeks of running and training and it leads to months, you can step it up. You won't be doing the ten minute walk or ten minute run and that sort of basic stuff that you started with; you're going to get better naturally.

That's what happens with baby steps: you get better, and then step it up a bit for a new, exciting challenge. Putting dates on these goals was important to know how much effort was needed for training.

The baby steps to achieve my goal to get back on my feet again, and walk after the stroke, started way back when I was lying in bed, with no control of my body in intensive care.

The baby steps were:

- being removed from intensive care into the ward
- gaining the ability to sit up in bed
- my speech coming back after ten days
- being able to get out of bed and into a wheelchair
- steering the wheelchair with my determined left arm
- daily rehabilitation with the OT team, to improve my right hand function
- daily physio sessions to learn to help me crawl again, and then kneel again
- standing with my physio's support
- walking side steps, hanging on a bar against the wall
- standing unaided
- getting a calliper for my leg
- walking forward with bars on either side to support me
- walking using a quad cane
- walking independently.

The Baby Step Method is simple – it's not rocket science! But there are people who haven't thought to use it to reach their big goal. Use it!

*Chapter 11 – Your Roadmap to the Finish Line*

## #training #lesson
## October 2013 – The big scary goal

The big day was here: 13 October, marathon day! I was expecting Shaun at my home at 4.30 am, so I planned to set my alarm at 3.30 am to get ready and prepare without panic. Maybe I ended up setting my alarm to 3.25 just to be sure!

Why was Shaun planning to come at 4:30 am anyway? I knew we needed to tape my left shin, but this was a ridiculous time for me. But surprisingly I was up for the Melbourne Marathon, chirpy and excited for a 3.25 am wake up call, and wasn't even nervous all week before.

Shaun planned to meet at my home, and then we were catching a train from a nearby station to avoid the hassle of finding a carpark. He turned up at ridiculous o'clock as promised; Chris arrived shortly after with a backpack loaded with energy balls and bits and pieces. I added a stash of jelly beans in small packs to this load, along with tissues. He kindly offered to carry my water bottle and blood glucose meter. I was planning to test my BG levels every hour as advised by my diabetes team. I'm sure we were over-packed; this was a marathon, not a three week hiking adventure! But at the time we felt that it was best to be prepared.

When preparing at home, I decided to wear a black armband to honour Brian. This was important to me, as he was one of the big reasons why I kept on this marathon journey. But to add to that, Shaun grabbed my wrist with a black marker in hand. 'What are you doing?' I asked.

'Donna, when I did my ultra-marathon in honour of my dad and granddad, someone wrote their names on my arm like this, and it was a good reminder to have in those tough times. Use this as motivation to keep going.' I smiled and agreed as he wrote 'BRIAN' inside my forearm. I probably didn't need it, but it was good to have, and it felt like Brian was with me.

It was time to go. We drove to the station in a cheery mood, all eager to go in the dark crisp cool air. We got to the train station to find it closed. Hmmm, maybe we were super-organised in every other area, but this was something I overlooked. So off we drove to the event and eventually found a carpark, still excited and in good spirits.

The crowd was buzzing, even in the cool fresh air. We found John, a fellow runner we'd arranged to meet, and we were a team of four in our Run Donna Run tops. This truly turned out to be bigger than I ever thought. An original idea of learning to run again, maybe a 4 km fun run as my personal challenge, had turned into a crazy marathon challenge journey that brought me here with an awesome running team – wearing Run Donna Run tops! John wasn't feeling the best though, he came down with a cold during the week before, but he was still committed and was there for the team.

John was an awesome man who contacted me after reading an article in a running magazine about my story. He was drawn to my story as his daughter, who was also a patient at the RCH, had only started walking again and faced

*Chapter 11 – Your Roadmap to the Finish Line*

challenges similar to mine. When he contacted me he said, 'How can I support?' I offered suggestions of donating or attending different fundraising events. He revealed he was a super-keen runner, and that he'd like to join our team on marathon day. So here he was! We formed a good friendship, and welcomed him with open arms. I had the pleasure of meeting his daughter Jess, who came to cheer us on, and I felt so blessed to have him on board.

An announcement was made over the loudspeaker, and it was time for all the runners to start heading for their positions at the start line – this was real now. We headed toward the start line and I saw Carla, my little sister, at the sideline shouting out to me. I ran up to her and gave her a big hug; as I ran off I heard her shout, 'Good luck!' I was so grateful that she came from Mildura, getting up so early to meet me there. I felt that I was already lucky.

Feeling like I was in a packed herd of excited and nervous sheep, I also felt the sense of excitement and a strange feeling in my gut, which I think is commonly called 'butterflies in the stomach'.

*Bang*! We were off and running!

The crowd of runners spread out eventually, allowing everyone to gain their own pace. I always felt better at running events when we spread out, and that's when the butterflies flew away. We weren't going fast for the guys' normal pace; when I apologised, Shaun grabbed my wrist and whacked it, promising he would do this every time I said sorry. We both smiled and kept moving.

Yes, of course there were plenty more 'sorrys' and whacks but I eventually learned. It wasn't a sunny day, but not overly cool ether – a good day for a long run. I knew this was going to be a long run, and was in good spirits. I had a huge smile thinking of how far I'd come.

Our first running buddy who joined us from the sidelines was Neil. He was wearing a Run Donna Run top that I gave him – awesome – and we were now a team of five. Neil always made me smile with his banter; he played a huge part in my journey as he, Shaun and the students from Shaun's college clinic treated me for the injuries that I faced during my journey. I think I was their unique class project, and I was very grateful for their treatment, support and smiles. He left us after spending about 5 km with us, and wished me well. I felt truly grateful for his support. Our team became four again.

As we kept moving, Chris kept up with reporting our pace and approximate time it would take us – timing was looking good. Both Shaun and Chris entertained us with their dad jokes. Then we came across another runner who was alone and looked like she was struggling a little. We ran beside her, introducing ourselves and checked to see if she was okay. Her name was Athena.

Shaun turned toward me and said without anyone else hearing, 'This is a sign, Donna!' I looked puzzled at him. 'The marathon originated in Athens, her name is Athena. We are running with Athena, it's a sign!'

I laughed as we kept moving and listened to Athena share her story.

She explained how she'd kept going to the 10 km mark, but was struggling now due to being hit by a car as she crossed the road, only a week before the marathon! So her next aim was the half-marathon mark, and maybe not completing the full marathon as she'd hoped to do.

Shaun explained my story briefly to her and asked if she wanted to join us. Our team then became five again. I was so inspired by Athena's determination and pleased to have an awesome addition to our team.

Shaun turned to me again. 'This is a sign, Donna!' I smiled at his enthusiasm and kept on our way.

Feeling a slight pain in my left hip, the old injury from the half-marathon crept up on me … not good timing. I tried keeping my pace with a grin, thinking, *Suck it up Donna, the power is in me!* 'The power is in me': the saying I used throughout the Run Donna Run journey, and even put on fundraising t-shirts, along with 'There's no such thing as can't'. It was something I even chanted at times when training; call me crazy, but it kept me moving forward and not dwelling on the pain.

I needed to walk at times … run, walk, run, walk, run and so on. I joked with Shaun that maybe he should have taped that awkward spot in my groin area, or maybe my whole body. We laughed as I tried to keep up good spirits with a grin, knowing that this was *not* going to be a short run in the park.

Going around a bend, I could see another runner in the distance running while waving and shouting, 'Run Donna, run!' Not recognising the woman, I waved and smiled; these moments really helped and also caught me by surprise at the same time.

We could see three other people waving up ahead on the right of the track; it was Thomas, Annitta and Laura, whom I originally met at the half-marathon challenge. Thomas was wearing his Run Donna Run top I'd sent him and a huge smile. I gave them all a hug and they ran with us. Our team had turned from five to eight keen people. We ran for a couple of kilometres together then said our goodbyes as Thomas, Annitta and Laura promised to meet us at the finish line.

Now back to our team of five, we saw a crowd of onlookers to the side as we came around the bend. We knew that I needed to stop soon for a BG test and a glucose gel. I saw my friends Neetha and Will with big smiles, standing there holding jelly snakes; I was so pleased to see them (and not just for the jelly snakes either).

This was proving to be an awesome day and a great example of how friends and even strangers who support and cheer you from the sidelines can really make a difference in helping you achieve great things.

After passing the crowd, we stopped at the sideline as I did a BG test. I was happy with the result but still took a glucose gel pack as advised by my diabetes team. We headed toward the beach road as it got cooler and windier, now even raining – this was not in the plan, but things don't always go as planned!

*Chapter 11 – Your Roadmap to the Finish Line*

We ran along the road where I lived and often trained, but this time on the road instead of the beach or path. I could see Carla yelling from the other side, with her boyfriend and my cousin Peter. It was raining and I was slowing down; I really wanted to get to Carla faster, feeling bad as they waited in the wind and rain for me. We were nearing the bend where I had to turn to get to the other side. I was feeling a deep pain; I had to walk for a while. It was now really cold and the rain was coming down fast.

We then spotted Rebecca, a friend, running toward us with her young daughter. They joined us and chatted for a while – the team became seven. I was amazed she waited in the rain and very grateful to see her at the same time; this made me smile, even if I was in pain. They left us after taking a few photos to put on social media. We said our goodbyes and picked up our pace again.

But the pain was now intense. Shaun got me to lay down on the side of the track as he worked his magic treatment on my hip, poking and prodding. It seemed to work, reminding me how great my team was.

We made it to Carla and Peter, both wearing Run Donna Run tops. She and her boyfriend ran 3 km with us. I was so proud of Carla. She had admitted being worried as she wasn't a runner, but wanted to support me, and proved to do both successfully. It was a great moment that I'll always be grateful for, to be running along with my little sis.

We neared the end of the road, where we turned around and passed Brian's path. I needed that moment to remind me of how far I'd come; it felt more significant with Carla and Peter beside me as we ran by Brian's path. I gave my keys to Carla for my apartment, so they could go and dry off. We said goodbye to Carla and her boyfriend as Peter stuck with us. We were now a team of six again.

We were well and truly past the half-marathon mark and I reminded Athena of how well she was doing, considering she was thinking of finishing her journey at the halfway mark. She kept telling me of how much I had inspired her; the feeling was very much mutual. I was so proud of her.

Now reaching the 28 km mark, I felt extreme pain on my left hip; this was the time where I really needed to dig deep. I felt that despite all the training and prep I had done, some things don't go as planned. Walking in the rain did not feel like a happy video time, as Shaun poked a cam in my face and told me to smile. I explained to him, 'You're not always going to get happy pics. '

'Talk to us, Donna.'

I turned and blew a raspberry at Shaun. 'Yeah, what do you want me to say?'

'Tell me what you're thinking.'

'Of the finish line.'

'What's it going to be like?'

'It's going to be an achievement.' Turning to

*Chapter 11 – Your Roadmap to the Finish Line*

Shaun, I added, 'I'm struggling a little bit right now.'

'That's okay. You've struggled before.'

'Yeah,' I said, agreeing with him.

'You know how to do that,' Shaun commented. I laughed.

Chris yelled out, 'We've reached the 28 km mark.'

'Only 14 km to go, you've done that plenty of times!' Shaun continued, trying to encourage me.

I laughed and said, 'Twenty-eight ks, woo hoo!' while groaning at the same time, and pushed on.

Shaun and Chris were always good at cheering me up and making me smile or laugh; I was truly grateful to have them on board, even though at first when they told me they were going to run with me on marathon day, I was initially nervous. The picture I had in my mind was of them both at the finish line, cheering me from the other side, but it was great to have them on my side all the way.

I kept soldiering on at a pace that I could manage, knowing that I had plenty more to endure. I said goodbye to Peter, to whom I was truly grateful for enduring the time and bad weather with us. We were now back to five.

It was now hailing and I felt that we had endured a pretty tough day. I turned to John, thanking him for joining us even with his cold – I was worried about him getting worse with this crazy weather, but he wanted to stay with the team all the way. He stated to me what an inspiration I was, and to keep thinking of the kids at the RCH. I nodded and smiled.

Moving further to my goal, I wasn't feeling good. Thinking I may have been low in my BG level, I suggested we stop and do a blood test.

Shaun said, 'I think you've got a few fans up ahead.'

I kept running and smiled, sucking it up. We could see a small group of people, two adults and three kids, holding banners in the rain. I didn't recognise them at first. As we got closer, I could see my best friend Carolyn from our university days, with her husband and three excited children. They'd all made banners and cheer pom poms, and I was so excited and grateful to see them, and they'd travelled from Mildura to watch me run! Wow! I wished I were in a better state, but also happy at the same time to see them. We said our goodbyes after our hugs and kisses and moved on.

We ran a little way and I did another BG test: it was good. This was me feeling the effects of the day at the 30 km mark, not a low BG level. I was reminded of the many marathoners I'd spoken to previously, who'd suggested that the 30 km mark was a spot where you either felt like you've hit the wall, or find your second wind.

Shaun handed me some chocolate and we kept going, still with Athena telling me how I motivated her. The rain stopped and it wasn't so windy; we kept going. My second wind came here. Or was it the reaction from the chocolate and Athena's kind words? I was so pleased we met her and that she stayed with us.

With only 10 km to go we then met Enisa, my diabetes educator, at the sideline with her husband. They joined us for a short time, Enisa asking me how I was going with my diabetes. I was so surprised and pleased to see her; I reported that my BG levels were on track. She left us with her gorgeous smile and encouragement as we kept on our journey.

My journey had been filled with so many encouraging and gorgeous people – not only on marathon day, but throughout the eleven months since the idea first came about.

Back to our team of five, we now needed to use the detoured route, as the roads were now open for the public. We followed the directions of the volunteers, and came across a woman who'd been running the marathon but had stopped and was hanging on to a pole on the side of the road, obviously struggling. Her friend was assisting her and motivating her to keep going.

'Oh, is she okay?' I thought aloud.

Shaun stopped to chat briefly and told her my story. As I kept moving, knowing she was in good hands, I could hear him behind me, chatting with her and giving his usual motivational speech that he gave me and all his clients, urging her to keep going. She followed us and kept going to reach her goal.

I turned behind me to say hi as she smiled and said hi back. Shaun yelled out, 'Donna, this is Tanya!' I was so inspired by her mind-shift and determination to keep going. This was gold to me. Our team became seven.

We stopped to use the toilet, with only 5 km to go. It was the first toilet stop I made all day. I knew we were so close to the MCG, but when a girl has to go, what can you do? So the whole team stopped, and we said goodbye to Tanya, our revived new friend, watching her keep going with her champion running buddy who had already completed the marathon but came back for her in her time of struggle – awesome stuff!

This marathon day was truly an inspiring journey in itself with the events, the people who joined us, the stories we heard and told – this was a day of extraordinary moments that captured my heart along the way.

Now with only 5 km to go, we were back to a team of five when Abbey, Chris's seven year old daughter, joined us to make a team of six. I felt so lucky to have so many join us that day, but at the same time would have liked to be in a better condition for when Abbey joined us. She was a trooper and smiled all the way, and I think Chris did too, being so proud of his daughter.

We then came across Kate, a workmate whom I really didn't expect to see. She always said at work she'd turn up as the 'orange girl', with orange wedges to keep me going, driving along beside me in a scooter – we would laugh about it all the time at work. But she actually came, in

*Chapter 11 – Your Roadmap to the Finish Line*

the terrible weather – without the oranges or scooter, but with support.

Getting closer to the MCG now! Shaun got a call from a friend with a camera in hand, letting us know there was very little time to get there before the MCG gates closed. Determined I would smash the doors open, I kept going with extreme pain – I wouldn't let them close the doors on me.

So this was not a 'world record speed' marathon challenge for me; I knew I wouldn't be the fastest, but this wasn't about speed for me. It was about endurance and getting to the finish line. Although I was a little annoyed, as the pace I began with before the hip injury crept back would have gotten me there quicker, I wouldn't let that overtake me now. I kept moving forward the best way I could, knowing that there were still others behind me whom I hoped would make it too.

Hobbling toward the gate, Thomas, Laura and Annitta were there as promised, Annitta running beside me and telling me what a great effort I'd put in. She revealed that her friend got injured and didn't make it to the finish line that day – he had to pull out. I was concerned but glad to hear he was okay now. She kept congratulating me and everyone cheered me on as I entered the MCG.

Entering the MCG in time, yay! I could hear the loud music and cheering in the distance. I was really struggling as Shaun whispered to me, 'Donna, this is your moment. Take it all in.' I heard my name over the speaker and the man's voice mentioned Run Donna Run; I wondered who had told him and laughed hearing it. Chris, John and Athena were still with me too, smiling as we entered. This was an awesome moment for me; even though I was still struggling with my hip, I had a huge smile thinking how far I'd come.

We were getting closer to the end and I could see familiar faces in the stand; I was surprised to see even a couple of my sponsors waiting in the crazy wet cold weather for me as well. It was awesome to see my family and friends all there in their Run Donna Run tops with 'There's no such thing as can't …' or, 'The power is in me!' printed on the front.

The rain stopped but the running track was still slippery from the rain. I asked Shaun as I was carefully running, 'Are you slipping? I think I'm going to slip on this track, are you finding it slippery? Or is it just me?'

I announced I would get off the track and run on the grass … the wet grass. Not thinking that they put a plastic track on the grass for a reason and the wet grass would be slipperier, I ran to the edge, hearing Shaun yell out, 'Nooo!' as he went to reach for my arm. It was too late. I landed face down, and for a moment my cheer squad went silent. I was only a few metres away from the finish line, I couldn't believe it! *OMG! Right here? Right now?*

Chris, John and Shaun came to rescue me and pulled me up – they were awesome. I felt like I was miraculously lifted off the ground without

*Chapter 11 – Your Roadmap to the Finish Line*

effort, as Shaun slapped my sun visor back on, saying, 'Go Donna!' I ran over the finish line with a huge smile, just making it in time.

This wasn't the same image I'd held in my mind as I trained for eleven months. I didn't imagine I would slip on the grass just metres before the finish line in front of everyone. I also thought I'd have a tear or two, maybe even a fist in the sky. But instead, I got up from slipping, got myself together again and back on the track. But I still ran with pride and relief over that finish line with a huge smile, turning to my team with kisses, hugs and gratitude for their awesome support.

I brushed the dirt off my legs from the fall, and announced to everyone with a grin, 'That was a bit of an embarrassing ending.'

Hearing chuckles but seeing tears in everyone's eyes. I gave a high five and hug to Athena and received my medal from Jess, John's daughter, which was awesome and an honour.

I looked up and was surprised to see everyone crying!

I turned to see my mum in front of me, giving me a huge kiss and hug and congratulating me. I didn't want to let her go, but then I saw my dad in one of my Run Donna Run tees. I was surprised (my dad doesn't wear t-shirts, ever) but he wore this to support me that day and had tears running down his face, saying how proud he was. Then more hugs from Carla, my aunty and cousins, other family from Mildura, my friends and sponsors, and people I met along the way.

My physio Julie was there too, waiting with a hug. We had reconnected a year before Run Donna Run and became good friends, so long since my lesson from her: 'There's no such thing as can't …' She wore the t-shirt too that day, saying just that.

I was so grateful for everyone waiting in the crazy weather to watch me reach my big goal. We took photos with family and friends, and my mum said to me, 'Brian would have been proud, Donna.'

I smiled. 'Thanks Mum.'

*'Success isn't how far you got, but the distance you travelled from where you started.'*
– Steve Prefontaine

Yes, I went through injuries, pain, heartache, blood, sweat and tears to reach that goal, but it was all worth it. That day changed my life, but the journey to get there changed me more so.

Are you ready to do the same and travel the distance to reach your big scary goal?

Are you ready to face the obstacles you may come across, the effort you need to put in? To get out of your comfort zone, and be able to pick yourself up again after the stumbles or slip-ups you may have?

If you answered yes to those questions and want to conquer your big scary goal, then it's time for you to make the move by using the Baby Step Method, which will give you the steps to reach your big goal. This applies to any goal!

Chapter 12

# The Baby Step Method

Creating your roadmap to your finish line is an individual process. Here I offer a simple Baby Step Method that I've used successfully myself and with others. But there are many ways to create individual plans for particular big goals to suit how each individual learns.

Go to http://rundonnarun.com.au/the-baby-step-method/ to print out your own Baby Step Method table. (See the diagram below for an example.)

When you have printed it, write your big goal at the top of the page, with your goal finish date. If you cannot think of an end date, seek a coach, mentor or simply use your own initiative.

For example: when do you want to leave your day job and start your business, to live a life you desire and change not just your life, but the lives of others? You need to be realistic with time, but I also I encourage it to be challenging too, if you want to reach it sooner rather than later. Remember you can simply change your date, if life gets in the way.

I suggest when you choose a date, say it is in eight months' time, set the date then break it down into doable timeframes. It could be monthly steps, so then it is broken down into eight baby steps. Eight doable steps.

You will have small steps now to consider on each line with an end date to each small step. 'I don't know where to start,' is a common response. Don't panic; start from the beginning of this book and keep it simple.

This can be scary, I know! I'm happy to help to get you started and on your track to success. Feel free to send me a message through http://www.rundonnarun.com.au/contact/ for further advice.

# The Baby Step Method (Example plan)

My big goal: *Run a Marathon, on 15 October 2017*

Baby step: (the step no. and describe or title it) *First Step – 5 km fun run*

I will achieve this on: (day, month, and year) *26 January 2017*

| Dates | Monday | Tuesday | Wednesday | Thursday | Friday | Saturday | Sunday |
|---|---|---|---|---|---|---|---|
| Week 1&2 | Walk/Run 20min | Rest day | Brisk Walk 20min | Walk/Run 20min | Rest day | 30-45 min | Rest day |
| Week 3&4 | Walk/Run 30–45min* | Rest day | Brisk Walk 30–40min | Walk/Run 30–45min | Rest day | 1 hour (as above) | Rest day |
| Week 5 | Walk/Run 30-45min* | Rest day | Walk/Run 30–45min | Walk/Run 30–45min | Walk/Run 30–45min | 90 min | Rest day |
| Week 6 | Walk/Run 30-45min | Rest day | Walk/Run 30–45min | Walk/Run 30–45min | Walk/Run 30–45min | 2 hour run | Rest day |

**Reward or celebration!** (Will it be at the end of each week? Will it be at the end of 4 or 6 weeks? Will it be when you achieve your step? You decide!) I will receive my medal on 26 January and go out for lunch with friends to celebrate.

\* or go longer if you feel ready.

## Notes:

- Saturday week 1-4 - 10min brisk walk, then 15-20mins run/walk, then walk for the rest of the time.
- Saturday week 5 & 6 trying to increase running time.
- Week 5 & 6 on Mon and Thurs – increase running time.
- Stretches every day!

Go to **http://rundonnarun.com.au/the-baby-step-method/** *to get your template to fill out your personal Baby Step Method plan for your goal.*

There are a few points with the Baby Step Method table that you'll need to consider to move forward and succeed in reaching your *big* goal.

- Repeat the process. Each format table is a baby step, okay? So it's up to you to make a few copies from http://rundonnarun.com.au/the-baby-step-method/, creating this format method again for your next baby step, and so on.

- This will be useful to take to your coach, mentor, or whoever you plan this with. Remember, each Baby Step Method table will be more challenging than the previous one. You may want to wait before creating your next table, as you'll find out from the previous table what worked well and what didn't, especially if you're new to the activities/commitments you write in your table.

- It is always good to review after each baby step; that's why journaling, writing or recording along the way is important.

- You will grow with each baby step and increase the intensity, forming a habit to get closer to reaching your awesome big goal.

- Make sure you start simple and make it fun, especially with your celebrations – they don't need to be big, fancy or expensive, but make them something to look forward to and relevant to your steps or big goal. It must be something you love and are looking forward to, not someone else's suggestion on what they think is a good reward or celebration. What will be your reward and motivation?

- Will your reward be at the end of each week? Will it be at the end of four weeks? How will you celebrate? Will the reward be an activity? Whom will you celebrate with? Will it be an item you buy for yourself? Write everything in the table. It could be every Sunday, or maybe you want to make it at the end of your four weeks – whatever you decide works best.

- Place your Baby Step Method table in a spot you will see every day. For example, the mirror, fridge, pin board or diary. It must be visible, and you must follow it to succeed.

Also note that *every* step format is individual for you and your particular goal. For example: the format for my marathon goal needed to have two 'rest days' spread out over the week, which was recommended by my expert coach. Ask your coach, mentor or someone you know who's achieved the same or similar goal. But don't get lazy with this either! If you want results, you need to be committed.

If you find you're a little stuck, please feel free to contact me at http://www.rundonnarun.com.au/contact/ and I will only be too happy to help achieve your awesome goal and reach your finish line.

Ready! Set! Go!

# Afterword

Congrats on reaching the end of this book, but this is not the end yet! This is only the beginning of your challenge; you are now at the start line with a great journey ahead.

What you can do now with your *big* goal dream is start your baby step plan. Make your individual plan that will work for you to reach your finish line. Refer to the table format of the Baby Step Method. Use it and make it work for your individual goal.

Be clear on what your big goal is. Write it down and stick it to your fridge door – or your wardrobe, your mirror, your car steering wheel – or even insert it into your computer screen saver … wherever you are reminded to see your goal every day! No 'if's' or 'but's' in this big goal statement either!

You need to think outside the box, and stop making excuses.

Another way to get around resilience is to think like a kid. People look at me odd when I say this. 'Think like a kid? What do you mean? I'm an adult! Why should I think like a kid?' Well, you've heard lots of people say how kids are just resilient, aren't they?

As an example, a friend of mine has a daughter who was diagnosed with a serious illness. Of course it was a big shock to family and friends.

I went to go and visit her. This was in the early days, when she was getting treatment. She had tubes attached to her, getting all the treatment that she needed; she was so happy to see me and she was chirpy with a big smile. It was awesome to see her. I sat beside her and asked how she was going. She'd tell me in a very matter-of-fact way, still with a smile and excited to see me, which was really nice.

I was asking her about what all these treatments were, and she knew what everything was: 'This is what they give me for this, this is what they give me for that.' At the same time she was forever smiling and grateful to have me as a visitor (and of course, other visitors coming along). She was super-inspiring.

But I remember when I left that visit and walked out of her room, I went up to her dad and said, 'She's amazing. She's in such good spirits, she's such a trooper.'

His reaction to me was, 'Yeah, kids are really resilient, aren't they?' And then he said to me, 'You'd know that, Donna.' I nodded and grinned.

The fact is that when we're kids, we think differently. People say to me even now, 'How did you get through that, with the stroke and then the diabetes?' It became my life, it was just normal after a while – well, not *normal*, but it was all that I knew. I did know the active and stroke-free body, of course, but it was just keeping on and pushing on, wanting to get better so I'd be able to do things with my friends, and my brother and sisters.

It's funny – this is something I don't even think my siblings are aware of. But growing up in my early years as the youngest child, I constantly wanted to be like my older brother, and especially like my two sisters. If they got their hair cut short, I wanted my hair cut short. When they were learning to play the organ and I was learning to play the guitar, I wanted to play the organ. Whatever they did, I wanted to do and be like them.

I may have seemed like the annoying younger sister, but I wanted to be just like them. This includes with their abilities too – sewing, art, even learning how to ride motorbikes with my brother. We were like your everyday siblings and would have our days where we'd argue, but they were there for me to look up to and strive to be like.

People often say, 'You're very determined, Donna.' I have my siblings to thank for that, as they were a reason *why* for me to keep going and be determined, as I wanted to be just like them.

Kids tend to get up if they stumble too and just keep going, have you ever noticed that? That's why I say to think like a kid!

Why aren't we doing this now? What has happened in between being a kid and growing up? We've grown up and all of a sudden we create these doubts in our mind and limiting beliefs; it's like something registers in our mind that takes away our confidence. But when you're a kid, it's like, 'Let's do it!' Without even questioning or doubting.

> 'At the end of the day, let there be no excuses, no explanations, no regrets.'
> – Steve Maraboli

The journey with my 'fellow soldier', my mother, did not end in 1979. Mum and I went to many appointments where rehabilitation was practised and repeated time after time. These appointments took me away from my classes at school, although this was a choice that needed no reasoning to my teacher.

There were so many visits to work with Liz, my lovely new occupational therapist in Mildura. She helped me strengthen my hand use and loosen the spasticity that formed with stubbornness and a stiff clenched fist; overcoming this was like a fight against myself.

Helen, my new joyful physio in Mildura, was another diligent appointment needed to get me walking independently without the need for the calliper, stick or wheelchair. I needed to develop strength and stability to stand alone, and walk without the need to reach out to catch my balance from the nearest object or person. The ability to pick myself up from a kneeling or seated position on the floor was among the tricks I previously took for granted.

We made visits to Mr Les, who applied remedial massage to my new awkward body.

After only a short time back at school, I collapsed in the schoolyard, shaking rapidly on the right side of my body. I felt as though someone was punching the right side of my body near my stomach, with me having no control of fighting this time. This was painful and scary.

Panicking, my school friends called a teacher and helped me to a bench to sit. What was happening? It eventually ceased; my mum was called and we went straight away to get medical attention.

These 'turns' were becoming a regular occurrence, varying in length of time and impact on my body. However, I was always aware of what was happening and felt the pain associated – it was exhausting. This was later described to me as a form of epilepsy, called a Jacksonian march, which I am pleased to say has been controlled for many years and is something I no longer experience! Another tough battle won!

There were other visits back to the RCH as well for regular check-ups with my specialists, who originally identified the critical condition of the Mystery Girl (now known as the Miracle Girl). They always greeted me with delight; these moments always reminded me of how lucky I am to have received such specialised attention and treatment. They always told me how glad they were to see me and how far I had come. I think they were even amazed!

Then there were other visits to the RCH to visit the diabetes department in my teens, with my new challenge of type 1 diabetes.

My parents and I became accustomed to long waits in patient waiting rooms at medical clinics.

I lived it! I came through, I survived and I fought with strength, determination, tears, laughs and motivation. I also had great support from everyone around me, whom I am dearly thankful for knowing and having in my life.

There are choices out there that we can make. Yes, there are times where we feel trapped in situations that we think we cannot control.

My belief is that we *can* control our decisions that we make.

I want to express that I do understand, from my own experiences, how we are sometimes caught in situations that we do not necessarily choose. I will use my own example of surviving a stroke as a young child, and type 1 diabetes as a teenager. I did not choose to be in that situation – of course not, nobody would! However, there are choices out there that we can make. When I say this I mean, how do we choose to handle our decisions, our life? Especially when also faced with challenges along the way.

I could have taken the road of feeling helpless or hopeless. I could have easily taken the sympathy of others and felt sorry for myself: the 'poor me syndrome'. I could have lost hope, lost the will, stayed on the gym mat crying, 'I can't, I can't!' and eventually gotten back in that wheelchair to let others do everything for me. But what sort of life would that have been for me? Or even more importantly, for my family and friends?

I choose not to be a victim!

I am not saying I am perfect – I am far from it!

There have been times that we can all relate to where our decisions take us along the more difficult, rocky, winding roads – rather than a smooth, sunny, drive-along easy road.

If you feel stuck in an unfulfilling job or career, where you feel stagnant, underpaid and unappreciated for your hard work and efforts, ask yourself: Is this my ideal job or employer? Is this how I see myself becoming happy, successful and financially secure? Is it in line with my goals and dreams? Am I waking up in the morning happy to be alive? Happy doing what I do? Happy being who I am?

Then there are other decisions that we make. Are we happy in our relationship? Is it fulfilling? Do I feel a deep connection with love, respect, emotional happiness and much more? Or is it a relationship that 'just is'? What can I do to improve my relationship? This is an area that I am certainly not an expert in, but these are choices also.

Health is another very important area of life. How am I treating my body? What am I feeding my body? Am I exercising? Do I feel physically good? How is this affecting my future? What can I do to improve my health?

Treat your body as your kingdom! Respect it. Nurture it, as we only have one body.

The people we surround ourselves with are very important for our growth and sanity. Are they people you choose to hang out with? Are your friends encouraging, respectful, fun, and supportive of your goals? Are you encouraging of theirs?

Sometimes we can get 'stuck' with friends that pull us down with negativity and sorrow. I am not saying to ignore your friends in times of struggles, not at all – but if this is becoming a habit of theirs, don't stay in that hole and that 'stuck' situation with them.

What I have learnt with my challenges along the way is that we are responsible for our own situation, positive or negative. There's no need to blame others or play the victim! This is only leaving it in someone else's hands, effectively letting go of your steering wheel.

It's okay to question, but why not get out of your comfort zone? When we stumble, just get up and keep going.

If you are feeling lost as to where to start:

- read this book again
- ask for help
- don't make excuses, find solutions
- get creative – think outside the box
- jump right out of your comfort zone,
- conquer the 'I can't' and adopt an 'I can' attitude

- push past the mental roadblocks
- understand that commitment gives power
- find your core why
- choose your distance
- get a training buddy
- celebrate the journey along the way
- use your winning language
- plan your road map
- learn resilience to get over the obstacle challenge.

I'm always super-excited to hear about people's journeys to their big goal, the thing that they've always dreamt about. I love the fact that they are willing to get off the couch and actually do whatever their big dream is, even if they know that it may be a difficult challenge. This is where these baby steps will definitely help you to achieve.

So feel free to contact me to let me know how you are doing at http://www.rundonnarun.com.au/contact/. I look forward to hearing from you, and cheering you from the sideline. I'm only too happy to help, if you need to get started with your plan. You can even let me know through social media how you are doing (see the links on the opposite page); I'd love to hear from you and find out what your *big* goal is.

Remember, the most important thing for you to get started, is for you to *believe you can* ... then make it happen.

Have an awesome time, now go conquer your big goals!

The power is in me ... and it's in you too!

*Afterword*

Keep up to date with Donna and her adventures at:

**Web**: www.rundonnarun.com.au
**Facebook**: www.facebook.com/RunDonnaRun
**Twitter**: @rundonnarun1
**Instagram**: run_donna_run
**YouTube**: Donna Campisi – Run Donna Run

# Acknowledgements

Writing this book has been a challenging time for me, but I'm used to challenges now. It has definitely brought back different emotions for me. I admit I've had times of tears through this journey of writing this book, for my family who have shown great strength and for other families at RCH who had their own challenges and losses ...

However, it has also given me smiles and chuckles in writing these memories of both struggles and successes, giving moments to reflect and offer you insights that I've gained along the way.

This journey has led me to a much brighter life than I could have ever imagined. I am able to inspire others now with my story, and I'm truly grateful to have met so many wonderful inspirational individuals along the way, who thank me for sharing my journey. This makes my heart glow.

There are a number of acknowledgements I'd like to make.

To my parents Nata and Vince. Even when speaking with my parents now about the testing time in 1978/79, they show complete solidarity in the strong faith and commitment they share. There were times they admit to doubting themselves, but they never lost their faith.

This is something that I haven't seen in all people and makes me truly grateful and honoured to have these two wonderful, strong people as my parents. You hear of parents saying how proud they are of their children at times – well, I am happy to declare how proud I am of my praiseworthy parents. They've taught me so much.

To Brian, Anne, Toni and Carla for their love, support and patience with me – for treating me like a 'normal' sibling, and inspiring me to keep determined. Much love and gratitude to you all. Including Madeleine, Conrad and Ren for your love and support too.

Thank you to Julie for teaching me, 'There's no such thing as can't …' and for our ongoing friendship. To the medical teams at the Royal Children's Hospital and later in Mildura for helping me get back on my feet, I am forever grateful.

This book is also for the unnamed in the RCH. Time can be made more fulfilling when filled with those around who give a simple hello, smile and nod. The laughter and the compassion that was shown all made a difference. To my visitors, my fellow roomies and their parents, and staff … everyone who entered my ward made a difference. Thank you.

To my wonderful friends who've kept encouraging me to keep writing – Kriss Oliver, Malka Silver, Sam Silver and Shaun Brewster – thanks heaps! I did it! Woo hoo! (Happy dance time).

Thank you Natasa and Stuart Denman, Blaise van Hecke, Kev Howlett, Les Zigomanis, Richard Burian, Tara Reid and the awesome Beau Hillier for your expert support, advice and skills in helping me get this book published and up and running (pun intended). You are all super encouraging and I truly appreciate you all!

A thank you to my awesome adventure hero Pat Farmer for your support, friendship and contribution in my Run Donna Run journey – and for the kind words written in my introduction. Thank you to Pat, Carol, Sabrina, Sam and Natasa for making the time to read and review my book.

To Enisa Kasar and the diabetes team at Baker IDI, thank you. T1Ds can do anything!

To my many enthusiastic and encouraging Run Donna Run followers, you rock! Your continued support has been tremendous and I will be forever grateful. And to those who ran with us on marathon day, you're all super awesome! Thank you!

Thank you to Justin Watts (from Sub4 Apparel) and Narelle Ash (from FlipBelt) who've supported me from the very beginning of Run Donna Run, and now give their awesome support with *The Unlikely Marathoner*. I appreciate your ongoing support and enthusiasm.

Thank you to Gene for planting the seed and encouraging me to write in the first place.

Shaun Brewster and Chris O'Driscoll, from Brewster's Running, thanks for your enthusiasm to come on board my crazy marathon journey. Your coaching, support, patience, treatments, commitment, dad jokes and obscure sayings made a difference, and meant a lot to me. I'm truly grateful. Thanks, BR Boys, for taking a risk and believing in me.

I kept going on my Run Donna Run journey and on marathon day because of my brother Brian. I've been asked whether there was a time I felt like giving up on marathon day. Not at all! That wasn't an option. He was a huge reason for me to keep on track. Brian was one of the first people I'd contact whenever something exciting or crazy happened on my marathon journey; his genuine enthusiasm was awesome and is greatly missed – He is greatly missed.

This book is written in honour of Brian: he was someone who always cheered me throughout my life from the sideline with my goals, big or small, and showed me what true courage is.

*The Unlikely Marathoner*
is proudly supported by our sponsors:

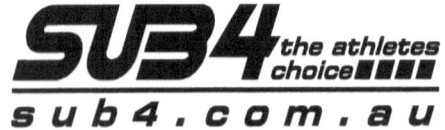

www.sub4.com.au

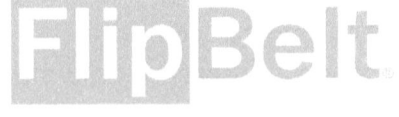

www.flipbeltaustralia.com

# About the Author

Donna Campisi is 'The Unlikely Marathoner'. She's faced big challenges throughout her life, including a stroke with other serious complications at seven years of age and being diagnosed with type 1 diabetes at fourteen.

After her stroke, doctors predicted that she would never walk or talk again. She was called 'The Mystery Girl' by the medical team because of her unusual symptoms.

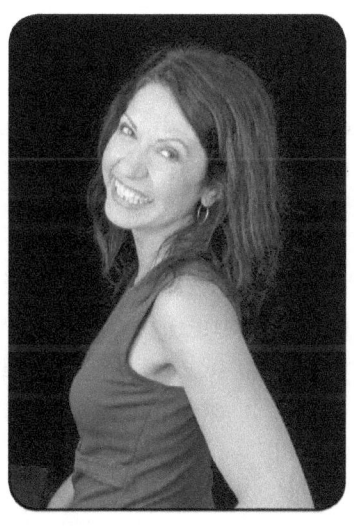

Donna's amazing recovery changed her name to 'The Miracle Girl.' But still, she had a long road ahead of rehabilitation, continually being pushed further out of her comfort zone.

An adventurer at heart, she now inspires many people with her 'can do' attitude through a campaign she created in 2012, called 'Run Donna Run'. Here, Donna certainly got out of her comfort zone, training from only being able to run thirty tentative steps in November 2012, to completing a marathon (42.2 km) in October 2013.

Run Donna Run began as a personal challenge to encourage other people to follow their dream, and spread her message that 'there's no such as can't' – a saying she learnt at a very young age when going through her own struggles to learn to walk again.

Run Donna Run became much bigger than she thought. She raised over $36,000 for the Royal Children's Hospital, which saved her life as a child, and went on to lead group adventure challenges and one-on-one coaching, which encourage people that they *can* actually do whatever they set their mind on, incorporating adventure and performance life coaching to gain results.

Donna's background includes studying and working in the disability field for people with intellectual, physical or mental conditions, where she learnt the benefits of baby steps. She then went on to study in training, presenting, life coaching and neuro-linguistic programming.

Today she is an inspiring speaker, marathoner, author, humanitarian, blogger, crazy runner, and adventure and performance coach. Inspiring many with her challenges and 'go do it' attitude, that they too are achieving their *big* scary goals!

Donna has a passion for supporting and fundraising for organisations in the community who need help also.

Donna is a contributor of the book *Inspirational Bible* and has also produced her own eBook, *Turn Dreams into Reality* – both can be found on her website below.

Donna is a woman who takes a challenge and believes it is achievable when broken into 'baby steps' and having the right mindset.

*About the Author*

You can keep up to date with Donna by joining her community at:

**Web:** www.rundonnarun.com.au
**Facebook:** www.facebook.com/RunDonnaRun
**Instagram:** @run_donna_run
**Twitter:** @rundonnarun1
**YouTube:** Donna Campisi – Run Donna Run

# Turn Dreams into Reality

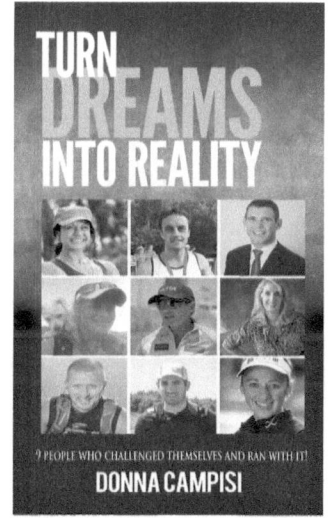

Donna's inspiring eBook 'Turn Dreams into Reality' is about 9 people who challenged themselves and ran with it. This book will certainly give you belief that anything is possible, even your own big hairy scary goal.

This inspiring book is about 9 everyday people who had their own huge dream and turned it into a reality.

Donna interviewed these people to share their insights on how they achieved their BIG scary goals, and became 9 extraordinary people.

'This inspiring book reveals how anyone can achieve their dream and turn it into a reality. If you need motivation and inspiration, this is a book for you.

Download your FREE copy here http://rundonnarun.com.au/free-ebook/

# Donna as a Speaker

Donna Campisi is an adventurer at heart. She's an inspiring speaker, author, blogger, humanitarian, crazy adventurer, and marathoner.

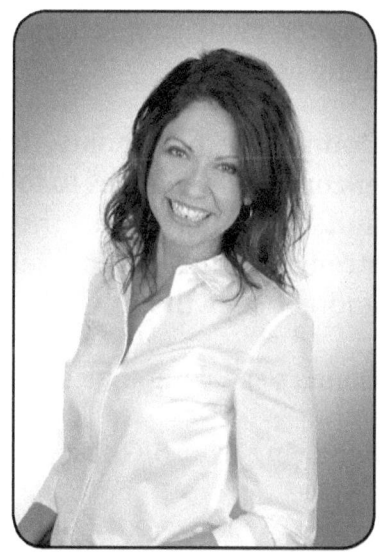

Donna is a highly skilled Adventure & Performance Coach. Inspiring many people with her group challenges and one on one coaching, and 'go do it' attitude, those who work with her are achieving their BIG goals!

Her message is to inspire and encourage others that 'there's no such thing as 'can't.'

She has proven this to be true time and time again! Doctors predicted Donna would never walk or talk again, and stated she was very lucky to be alive after surviving a stroke and other serious complications at 7 years of age. She is very much alive, walking and talking! At 14 years of age, Donna faced another challenge and was in another critical condition, diagnosed with type 1 diabetes.

In November 2012, Donna created her own major challenge, inspiring many people along the way. Only able to run 30 tentative steps in Nov 2012, she challenged herself to complete a marathon in October 2013. Creating her own campaign called 'Run Donna Run', she raised over $36,000 for the Royal Children's Hospital Foundation.

Donna is a woman who meets a challenge head on and believes it is achievable when broken into 'baby steps', along with having the right mindset. She shares with confidence "Don't just take opportunities when they come along. Create opportunities!"

Since completing her marathon challenge, Donna has inspired many people around the world, that there's no such thing as 'can't'.

**Donna is a passionate, inspiring woman, who aims to encourage audiences to follow their dreams, and succeed, and to bring back their confidence, independence, strength, courage and self-belief that they CAN achieve and get over the finish line.**

Donna's speaking topics include:

Achieving your BIG scary goals:

- Creating Your Baby Step Plan
- Steps to reach your big goal
- How to get to your finish line

There's no such thing as can't ...

- The Resilience Factor
- Finding your WHY
- Think like a Kid.

Boosting Your Confidence to Achieve

- How are you selling yourself?
- Women in business
- The Power is in ME! – the power of choice

Donna can adapt her inspiring story to a topic of your choice.

Her contagious positive attitude and highly engaging manner bring warmth, laughter and a mix of emotions to an audience when hearing her speak leaving them motivated and inspired to believe anything is possible.

Contact Info:

    www.rundonnarun.com.au/contact/

    www.rundonnarun.com.au/speaking/

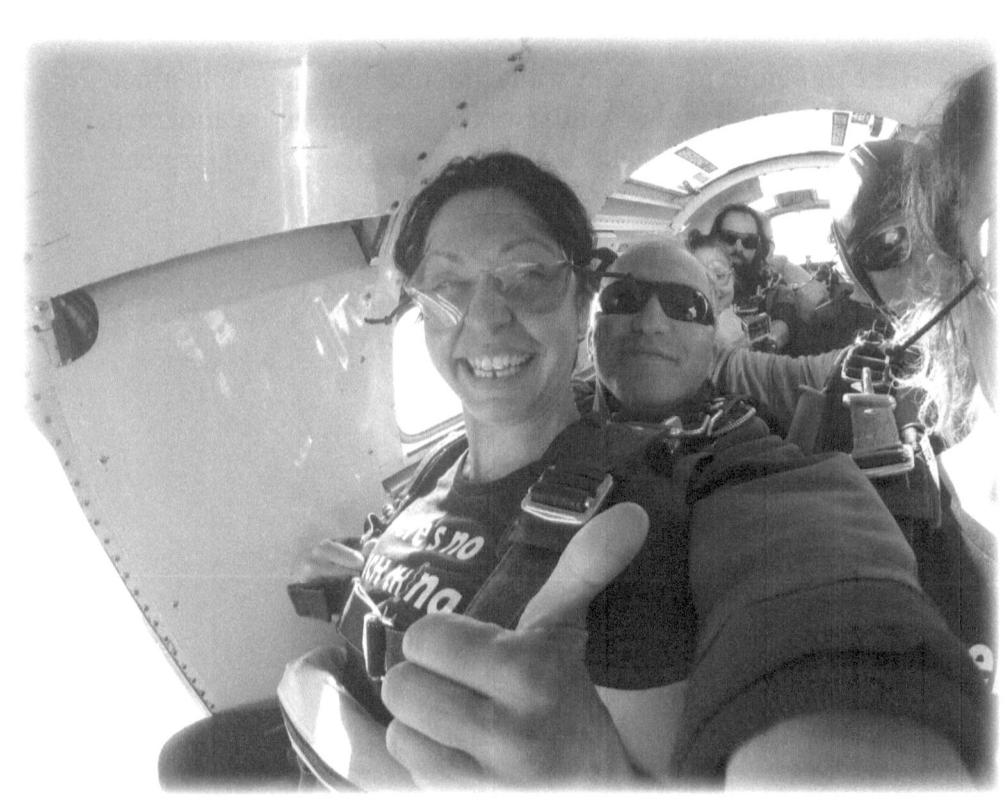

# ADVENTURE BEYOND LIMITS

### We are ABL

We are ABL to reach our BIG goals, by facing challenges to get you over your finish line.

Donna holds adventure programs that will excite you, push your limits, get you out of your comfort zone, and give you confidence. You will gain courage, self-belief, clarity, resilience and determination to achieve anything!

These programs have changed lives, and given results that have even shocked our participants ... for the better!

Donna's adventure programs include BIG challenges such as:

- Running challenges
- Hiking adventures
- Skydiving
- Hang-gliding
- And more coming up ...

Participants gain confidence to do bigger goals in their life, whether it be for work or play!

To find out more about our current Adventure Beyond Limits programs, contact Donna at www.rundonnarun.com.au/contact/ to discuss your goals.

"Donna's program was the best thing I have ever done to improve my health and lifestyle. It was a well-supported holistic approach to running, suitable for any level of fitness. When I joined the program I was recovering from serious health issues and had only returned to work four months earlier after six months sick leave. The flexibility of the program, the constant online support and excellent graduated training and nutritional information was the key to the success. My friends and family were amazed at my progress and success. I would highly recommend this program to my family and friends."

    Julie Buick,
    *Paediatric Physiotherapist, Chelsea*

"Overall it was a great experience which had plenty of laughter, support, strength and challenges. I wouldn't have been able to train myself to run 15km nor would I want to. Donna's program was a fun way of training and pushing myself to do more. It was great to make running a team effort and have everyone learning together and encouraging each other."

    Sarah Smith,
    *Senior Travel Consultant, Mildura*

"I just went for a RUN!! OMG I can't believe that I actually woke up and felt a desire to go for a run! The usual voices in my head that tell me it will be too hard were still there, but my body just kept getting my running gear on as they chattered away. Something has shifted! Just spending time with Donna gave me that thing, I have never experienced. I DID IT!! So proud and happy with myself right now!"

    Kelly Vanyai
    *Coach and Mentor, Gold Coast*

"I wouldn't have believed I could actually run 15km, ever: but I did. It is great to have the support of everyone on the Facebook group, and it was actually good that I didn't know anyone prior to starting. I am normally a very private person but was able to be much more extroverted on the group page. And I think I have made some friends for life through it. The number one thing I learnt from this program, is that I can do things that I didn't think I could. And that some other people find running as difficult as I do! It did put me outside my comfort zone, and there were a couple of challenges I thought I wouldn't enter that I did at the last minute. Sticking to the program for 20 weeks was the toughest challenge that I completed! They kept me accountable because I was reporting back and hearing what others were doing too."

**Joanna Maidment**
*Secondary Teacher, Rosebud*

"The program had a group of fun, positive, inspirational, motivated, supportive people with a great sense of team ship. It also had expert advice in sports injury prevention and treatment, running programs, sports nutrition and general health and nutrition. There were also great competitions and prizes. The challenges I thought were all great, I'd do them all as they have a varied group who would have diverse tastes, so there was something for everyone."

**Laura Scott**
*Dalmore*

# Notes

# Notes

# Notes

# Notes

# Notes

www.ingramcontent.com/pod-product-compliance
Lightning Source LLC
Chambersburg PA
CBHW021147080526
44588CB00008B/246